BLOW AWAY THE PULMONARY BOARDS...

Questions You Must Know to Pass the Exam

Jeremiah S. Reedy MD

CONTRIBUTING AUTHORS **Andrew Sherrick MD & Chad DeFrain MD**

ISBN 10: 1493642952
ISBN 13: 9781493642953

To Brenda, for tolerating the countless hours I've spent studying for Board exams over the years.

JSR

TABLE OF CONTENTS

Audience

- Pulmonary medicine fellows preparing for the American Board of Internal Medicine certification examination in pulmonary medicine.
- Pulmonologists preparing for the American Board of Internal Medicine maintenance of certification examination in pulmonary medicine.

Objectives

- Assess current knowledge in pulmonary medicine.
- Strengthen core knowledge of material relevant to the certification or recertification examinations.
- Identify subjects that may need to be further studied or improved upon prior to taking the certification or recertification examinations.

Financial Disclosure

None

Staff

Author and Editor:
Jeremiah S. Reedy, MD
Central Illinois Allergy and Respiratory Services
Clinical Assistant Professor
Southern Illinois University School of Medicine
Springfield, Illinois
Contact: Support@Blowawaythepulmonaryboards.com

Contributing Authors:
Andrew Sherrick, MD
Clinical Radiologist, S.C.
Professor of Medicine
Chairman, Department of Radiology
Southern Illinois University School of Medicine
Springfield, Illinois

Chad DeFrain, MD
Medical Director, Clinical Chemistry and Toxicology
Memorial Medical Center
Clinical Assistant Professor
Southern Illinois University School of Medicine
Springfield, Illinois

Acknowledgements

- Carla Cox and Diane Sample for assistance with manuscript preparation.
- Julie Brown and the medical library staff at St. John's Hospital and Memorial Medical Center in Springfield, IL, for assistance in gathering reference material.

Notice

Medicine is an ever-changing science. While every effort has been made to ensure the accuracy of the information provided in this book, changes in medical practice and drug therapy occur rapidly. The content in this book is designed to assist with preparation for the American Board of Internal Medicine certification and maintenance of certification examinations in pulmonary medicine and not for clinical practice. Users of this book are encouraged to consult other resources for all aspects of patient care. The authors do not assume any liability for any adverse outcome that may occur as a result of using the material in this book. The authors do not guarantee a passing score on either the certification or the maintenance of certification examinations in pulmonary medicine.

ABBREVIATIONS

Acute eosinophilic pneumonia	AEP
Acute interstitial pneumonitis	AIP
Acute respiratory distress syndrome	ARDS
Adenosine deaminase	ADA
Allergic bronchopulmonary aspergillosis	ABPA
Amyotrophic lateral sclerosis	ALS
Antineutrophil cytoplasmic antibody	ANCA
Antinuclear antibody	ANA
Benign asbestos pleural effusion	BAPE
Chronic eosinophilic pneumonia	CEP
Chronic obstructive pulmonary disease	COPD
Chronic thromboembolic pulmonary hypertension	CTPH
Community-acquired pneumonia	CAP
Confusion, urea, respiratory rate, blood pressure	CURB
Cryptogenic organizing pneumonia	COP
Cyclooxygenase-1 inhibitor	COX
Cystic fibrosis	CF
Cystic fibrosis transmembrane regulator	CFTR
Deep venous thrombosis	DVT
Deoxyribonucleic acid	DNA
Desquamative interstitial pneumonitis	DIP
Epstein Barr virus	EBV
Exercise-induced bronchospasm	EIB
Forced expiratory volume in 1 second time	FEV_1
Forced vital capacity	FVC

Gastroesophageal reflux	GER
Granulocyte macrophage-colony stimulating factor	GM-CSF
Hepatopulmonary syndrome	HPS
Hereditary hemorrhagic telangiectasia	HHT
High efficiency particulate air	HEPA
Human immunodeficiency virus	HIV
Hypersensitivity pneumonitis	HP
Idiopathic pulmonary fibrosis	IPF
Laryngopharyngeal reflux	LPR
Lupus erythematosus	LE
Lymphoid interstitial pneumonia	LIP
Noninvasive positive pressure ventilation	NIPPV
Nonspecific interstitial pneumonitis	NSIP
Obstructive sleep apnea	OSA
Polymerase chain reaction	PCR
Posttransplant lymphoproliferative disorder	PTLD
Primary ciliary dyskinesia	PCD
Provocative concentration in mg/mL causing a 20% fall in FEV_1	PC_{20}
Pulmonary alveolar proteinosis	PAP
Pulmonary arterial venous malformation	PAVM
Pulmonary embolism	PE
Reactive airway dysfunction syndrome	RADS
Systemic lupus erythematosus	SLE
Transfusion-related acute lung injury	TRALI

SUBJECT INDEX

QUESTIONS

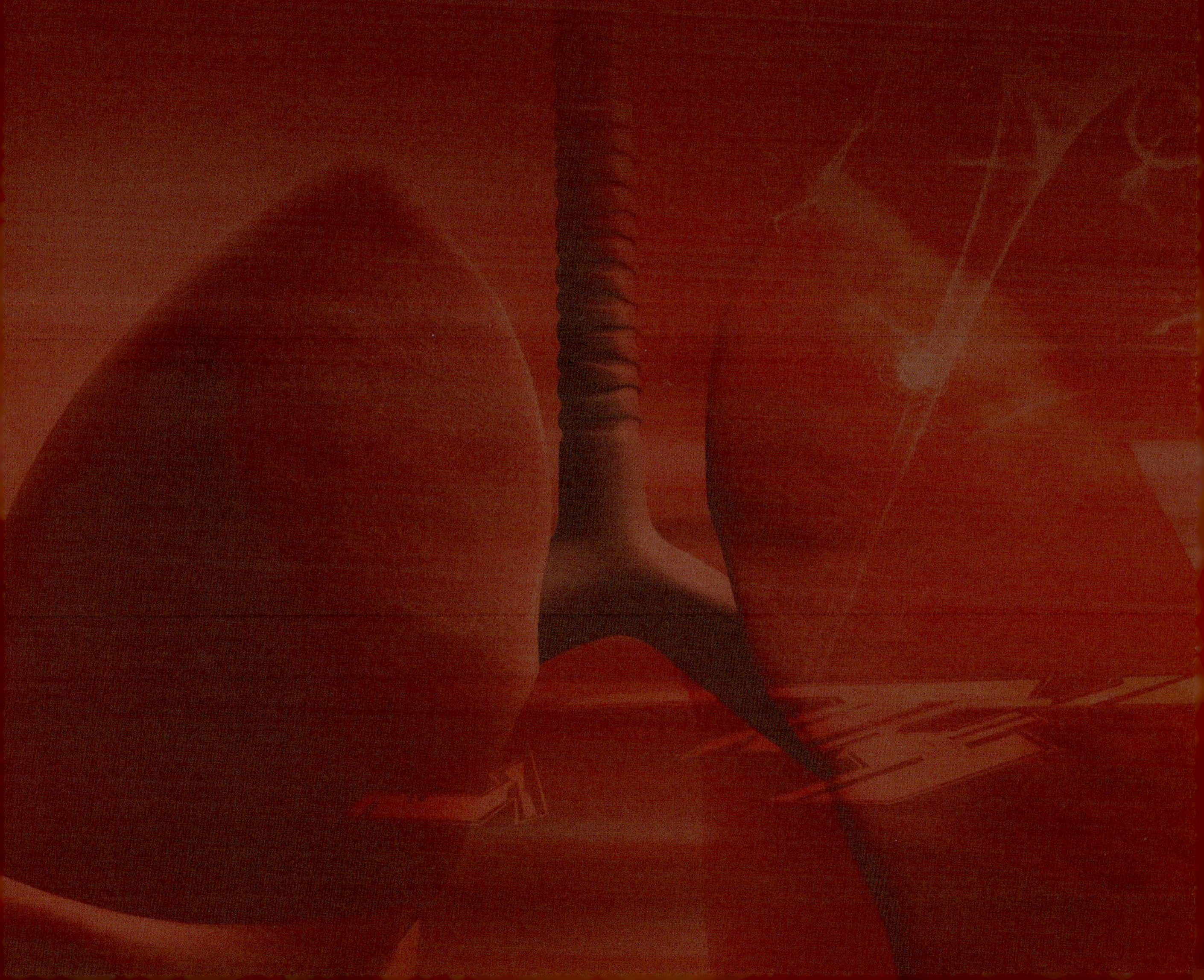

1. A 57-year-old female presents with a dry cough, fatigue, malaise, and a 14-pound weight loss. On physical examination temperature is 36.6°C, heart rate is 62 beats/min, blood pressure is 119/62 mm Hg, and respiratory rate is 18 breaths/min. Inspection of the thorax is notable for retraction of the inferior sternum and xiphoid process. Cardiac examination reveals a high-pitch, late systolic murmur. Midinspiratory and expiratory crackles are present throughout both lungs. High-resolution computed tomography scanning of the chest is performed. Representative images are shown in figures 1-A and 1-B.

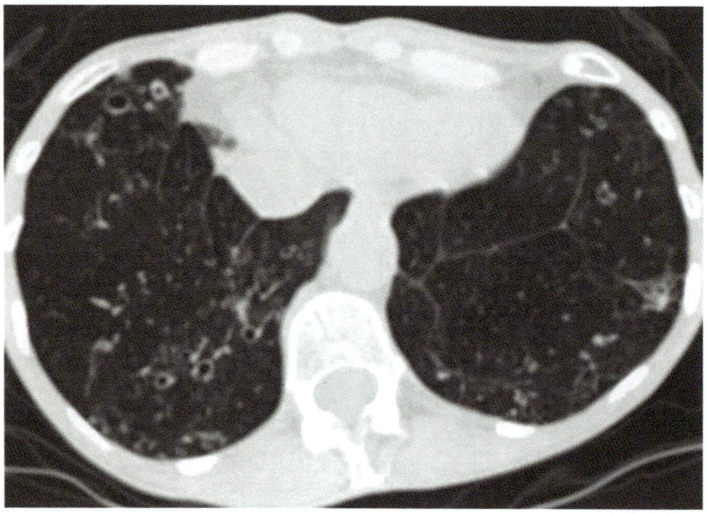

Figure 1-A

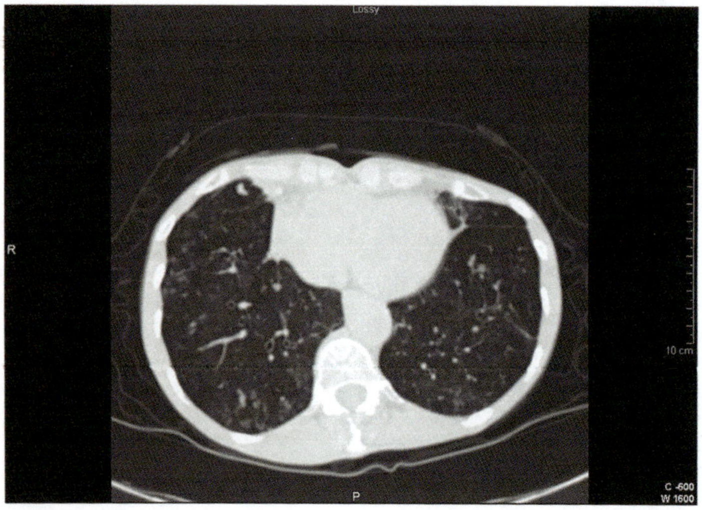

Figure 1-B

Which one of the following would not satisfy the microbiologic criteria for diagnosing a nontuberculous mycobacterial lung disease?

A. Two out of three separate expectorated sputa samples are culture positive.
B. A single positive culture is obtained from a bronchial wash.
C. A single transbronchial biopsy reveals granulomatous inflammation with acid-fast bacilli present.
D. A single transbronchial biopsy shows granulomatous inflammation. An expectorated sputum is culture positive.

2. Which one of the following statements about reactive airway dysfunction syndrome is true?

A. Can occur following a single exposure to a low level of a toxic substance.
B. Most individuals have a history of atopic disease.
C. Respiratory symptoms usually do not persist for more than a few weeks following the time from initial exposure.
D. Individuals may return to the workplace/environment and be re-exposed to low levels of the causative agent without becoming symptomatic.

3. A 56-year-old female is undergoing evaluation for worsening shortness of breath and a nonproductive cough. She was in her usual state of health until several months ago when symptoms gradually developed. She is a lifelong nonsmoker. Past medical history is remarkable only for dental cares. She is on no prescription medications. A review of systems is positive for dry eyes without any loss of vision and fatigue.

On physical examination the patient is in no distress. Vital signs are stable. Ocular evaluation is notable for bulbar conjunctival vessel dilation bilaterally. Examination of the oral cavity shows gingival recession. Cardiac examination reveals a regular rhythm without any murmurs or gallops. No adventitious sounds are appreciated with auscultation of the lungs. Digital clubbing is not present. Westergren erythrocyte sedimentation rate is 36 mm/hour. Antibodies to double-stranded DNA are 10%, IgG anticardiolipin antibody is 15 GPL, antimitochondrial antibody is 1:3, C3 is 200 mg/dL, and C4 is 32 mg/dL. Posteroanterior and lateral view chest radiographs show patchy interstitial and alveolar opacities. High-resolution computed tomography scan of the chest shows areas of ground glass opacities and consolidation throughout both lungs.

The patient undergoes video-assisted thoracoscopic biopsies of the right upper, middle, and lower lobes. A representative image is shown in figure 3-A.

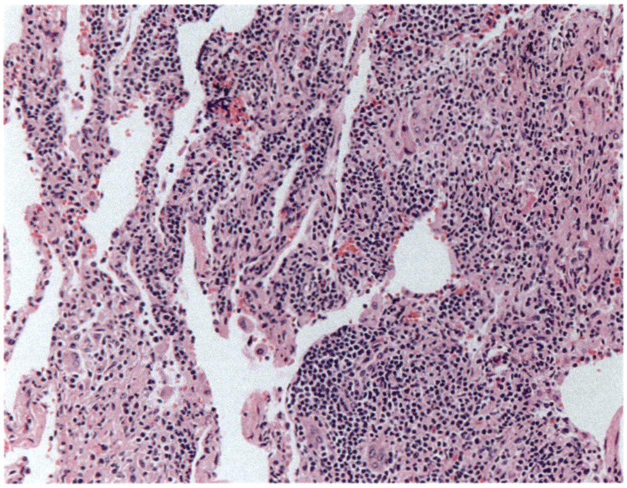

Figure 3-A

Which one of the following statements about this condition is true?

A. Malignant transformation is uncommon.
B. The interstitial lymphoid infiltrate is comprised mostly of B-lymphocytes.
C. Immunophenotyping of lymphocytes obtained from bronchoalveolar lavage fluid will show clonality.
D. Progression to end stage fibrosis and death will occur.

4. A 70-year-old female with a history of chronic obstructive pulmonary disease is being discharged from the hospital following an acute exacerbation. This is her 3rd hospitalization in the last 2 months. She is being discharged on a tapering dose of prednisone. In addition, she is taking tiotropium one inhalation daily, budesonide/formoterol 160/4.5 mcg two inhalations twice daily, roflumilast 500 mcg orally once daily, furosemide 40 mg orally once daily, and albuterol administered by a nebulizer every 4 hours if needed. She uses supplemental oxygen 4 L/min continuously. She has a pressure preset noninvasive positive pressure ventilator that she uses when sleeping.

The patient has an approximately 100-pack-year history of smoking cigarettes and despite efforts to remain abstinent, still consumes close to half a pack of cigarettes per day. The most recent FEV_1 was 18% of predicted with no response to bronchodilators. Past medical history is notable for nonocclusive coronary artery disease, chronic kidney disease, and cor pulmonale. Computed tomography scanning of the chest obtained during this hospitalization shows a homogenous distribution of emphysema bilaterally. An alpha-1antitrypsin phenotype is MZ with a plasma level of 16 micromole/L.

Which one of the following should be performed next?

A. Enroll in hospice.
B. Weekly intravenous administration of pooled human alpha-1 antiprotease.
C. Pulmonary rehabilitation followed by lung volume reduction surgery.
D. Pulmonary rehabilitation followed by single lung transplantation.

5. A 62-year-old male is being evaluated in the emergency room after developing sudden shortness of breath. He also complains of diffuse chest pain worse with deep inspiration. He had a right total hip arthroplasty 4 weeks ago. He received perioperative fondaparinux for prevention of venous thromboembolic disease for 10 days. On physical exam the patient is in moderate distress and appears anxious. Respiratory rate is 29 breaths/min, heart rate is 135 beats/min, blood pressure is 135/90 mm Hg, and temperature is 38.2°C. Jugular venous pulsations appear normal. Auscultation of the lungs reveals a continuous squeaky noise over the right 5th intercostal space. Friction fremitus is present over this area. Mild edema is noted in the right lower extremity. The surgical incision site is unremarkable. A portable anteroposterior chest radiograph shows a nonspecific density in the right lower lobe. A stat ventilation profusion scan is obtained and shows a large segmental-size mismatched defect in the right lower lobe.

Treatment with a continuous infusion of intravenous unfractionated heparin using a weight-based dosing protocol is initiated in the emergency room. A short time later the patient's condition markedly deteriorates. Repeat vital signs show a respiratory rate of 32 breaths/min, blood pressure of 80/40 mm Hg, and heart rate of 160 beats/min. Oxygen saturation recorded by continuous pulse oximetry is in the mid-80% range on 2 L/min of supplemental oxygen administered via a nasal cannula. A bedside echocardiogram is obtained.

Which one of the following would be an indication for the administration of intravenous thrombolytics?

A. Severe pulmonary hypertension identified on the echocardiogram.
B. Presence of a large mismatched defect on ventilation-perfusion scanning.
C. Hypoxemia.
D. Systemic hypotension.

6. A 38-year-old female is found on routine preemployment chest radiographs to have a rounded, noncalcified mediastinal mass. She denies chest pain, cough, shortness of breath, hemoptysis, and fever. She has a 5-pack-year history of smoking cigarettes. Physical examination is unremarkable. Computed tomography scanning of the chest with intravenous contrast is performed. A representative image is shown in figure 6-A.

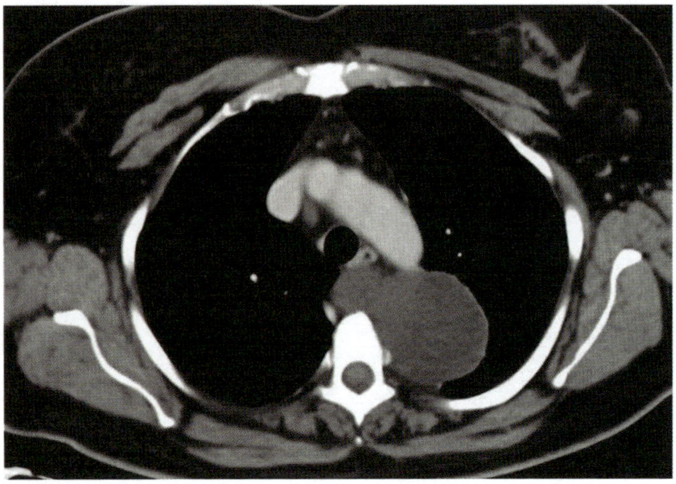

Figure 6-A

Which one of the following should be performed next?

A. Thoracotomy with surgical resection.
B. Transbronchial fine needle aspiration.
C. Percutaneous fine needle aspiration.
D. No further evaluation is indicated because the radiographic features are consistent with a benign process.

7. Which one of the following statements regarding minute ventilation during normal pregnancy is true?

A. There is an increase in minute ventilation as a result of an increase in respiratory rate.
B. There is an increase in minute ventilation as a result of an increase in tidal volume.
C. There is an increase in minute ventilation as a result of an increase in both respiratory rate and tidal volume.
D. There is no change in minute ventilation.

8. A 35-year-old female presents with pain in both ankles and a rash on her right leg. She was well until a few weeks ago when she noticed discomfort in both ankles. She doesn't recall any trauma. She denies involvement in other joints. She then developed a painful lesion on her right leg. Over time, the area evolved into a bruise. A review of systems is positive for the sensation of a low-grade fever. Inspection of the skin overlying the right pretibial area shows an approximately 2 cm violet-colored nodular lesion. It is tender to palpation. There are no other cutaneous findings. Examination of the ankles shows no soft tissue swelling, evidence of effusion, tenderness, erythema, or warmth. A full range of motion is present. Cardiopulmonary examination is unremarkable. Chest radiographs are performed and shown in figures 8-A and 8-B.

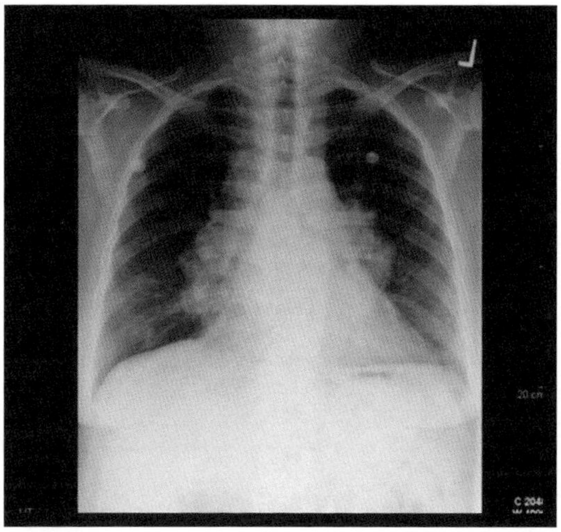

Figure 8-A

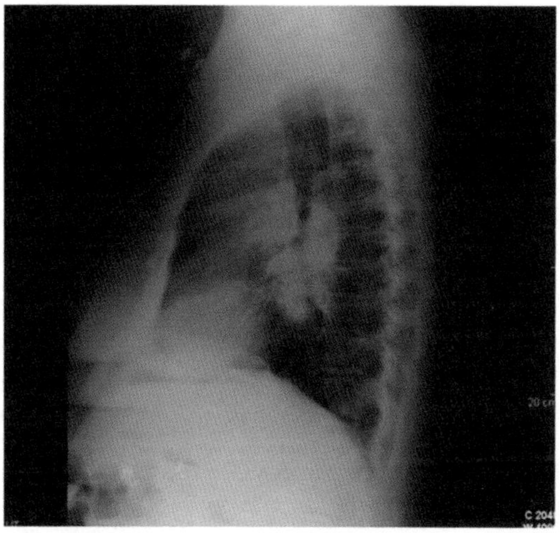

Figure 8-B

Which one of the following statements about this condition is false?

A. It will most likely spontaneously remit.
B. Skin biopsy will show tight, well-formed caseating granulomas.
C. Iritis and facial palsy can complicate the course.
D. An angiotensin converting enzyme level is almost always normal.

9. A 36-year-old nonsmoking male presents with a low-grade fever, worsening shortness of breath with exertion, and a cough productive of brown sputum. Past medical history is positive for asthma since early childhood. He recently completed a prolonged course of prednisone for a similar illness. He works as an assistant editor for a locally published newspaper. There are no pets in his home and he reports no recent travel. Current medications include fluticasone/salmeterol 500 mcg/50 mcg one inhalation twice daily, montelukast 10 mg orally once per day in the evening, and rescue therapy with an albuterol metered dose inhaler two inhalations every 6 hours as needed.

On physical examination temperature is 37.9°C, respiratory rate is 20 breaths/min, heart rate is 102 beats/min, and blood pressure is 134/82 mm Hg. Inspection of the thorax shows no chest wall deformities.

Auscultation of the lungs demonstrates a prolonged expiratory phase and monophonic wheezes bilaterally. Leukocyte count is 10,000/cu mm with 10% eosinophils. Serum IgE is 2,036 IU/mL. Computed tomography scanning of the chest is performed. A representative image is shown in figure 9-A. A skin prick test for *Aspergillus fumigatus* antigen is immediately positive. His peak flow is decreased 250 ml from baseline.

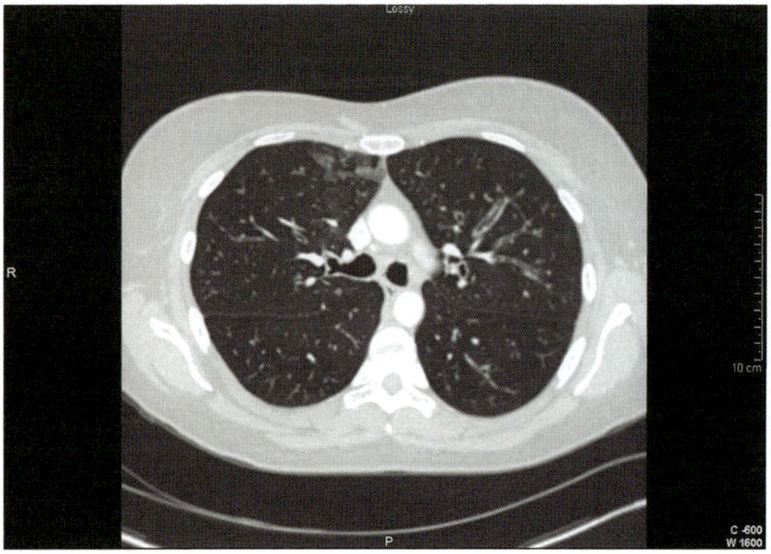

Figure 9-A

Which one of the following treatments should be recommended?

A. Omalizumab.
B. Itraconazole.
C. Inhaled fluticasone.
D. Prednisone and itraconazole.

10. A 75-year-old male with severe chronic obstructive pulmonary disease enrolls in a pulmonary rehabilitation program. Participation in pulmonary rehabilitation has been shown to lead to all of the following except which one?

A. Improvement in the symptom of dyspnea.
B. Increase in survival.
C. A reduction in the number of hospitalization days for acute exacerbations.
D. An overall decrease in health care utilization.

11. A 43-year-old-male with a body mass index of 34 kg/m^2 presents with a complaint of shortness of breath that is worse with physical activity. He has no history of lung disease. Chest radiographs are unremarkable. He is a nonsmoker.

Pulmonary function testing is likely to show all of the following except which one?
A. Normal expiratory reserve volume.
B. Normal residual volume.
C. Normal ratio of the forced expiratory volume in one second to forced vital capacity.
D. Normal diffusing capacity.

12. Which one of the following statements about methotrexate-induced hypersensitivity pneumonitis is false?
A. A skin rash may be present.
B. Blood eosinophilia is common.
C. Hilar and mediastinal adenopathy can occur.
D. Despite drug withdrawal, the majority of patients will have residual chronic fibrosis.

13. A 44-year-old male presents with several months of progressive shortness of breath and cough. A review of systems is negative for fever, chills, night sweats, chest pain, and weight loss. He has a 30-pack-year history of smoking unfiltered cigarettes. After high school he briefly served in the navy for 2 years. He is currently a certified public accountant. He reports no recent travel history or tuberculosis exposure. He is not on any prescription medications.

On physical examination the patient is afebrile. Respiratory rate is 22 breaths/min. Oxygen saturation measured by pulse oximetery is 86% while breathing ambient air. There is a faint, bluish discoloration about the ears, lips, and nail beds. Digital clubbing is present. Expansion of the thorax is normal. Auscultation of the lungs reveals bronchovesicular breath sounds over the upper interscapular area and early-to-mid fine inspiratory crackles at the bases. Pulmonary function test shows a total lung capacity of 76% of predicted and a diffusing capacity of 64% of predicted. Chest radiographs shows vague lower lobe opacities. Computed tomography scanning of the chest is performed. A representative image is shown in figure 13-A. A thoracoscopic lung biopsy is performed. A representative image is shown in figure 13-B.

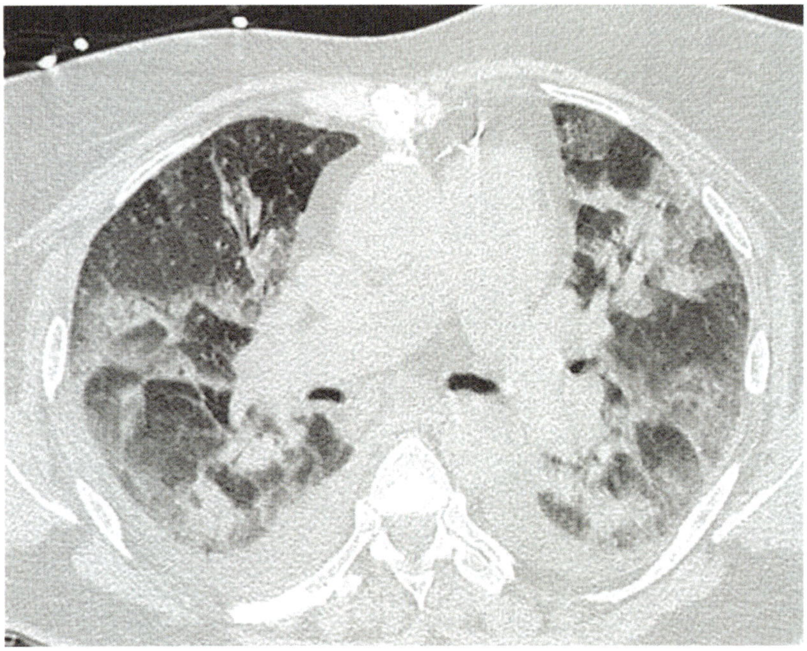

Figure 13-A

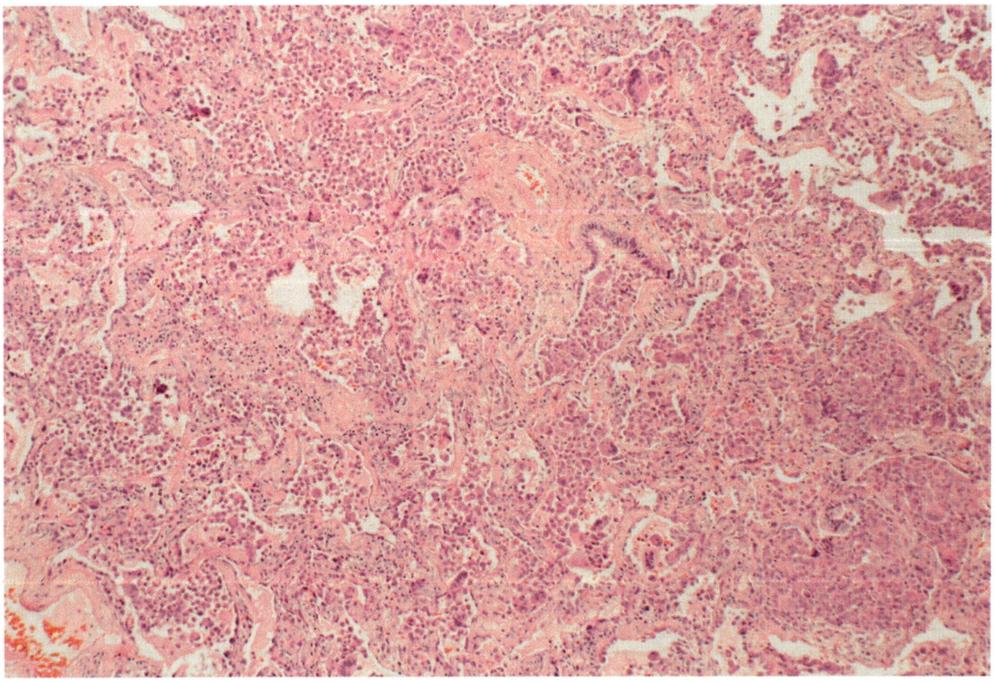

Figure 13-B

Which one of the following statements about this condition is true?
A. Mean survival is similar to that of patients with usual interstitial pneumonitis.
B. The majority of cases occur in cigarette smokers.
C. Males and females are equally affected.
D. Honeycombing with traction bronchiectasis will eventually develop.

14. A 24-year-old male is evaluated in the emergency room in the month of July for an acute febrile illness. He also complains of headache, malaise, nonproductive cough, shortness of breath, and chest pain. Symptoms began several days after working on a farm property at Martha's Vineyard. He denies handling any rabbits, skunks, or raccoons, but did participate in activities such as lawn mowing and brush cutting.

On physical examination the patient appears acutely ill. Temperature is 38.6°C, heart rate is 89 beats/min, blood pressure is 136/74 mm Hg, and respiratory rate is 28 breaths/min. Conjunctivae do not appear inflamed. Oropharynx is moist without any exudates. There is no cervical, axillary, or inguinal adenopathy. Abdominal exam does not reveal any masses or organomegaly. There are fine inspiratory crackles in the left lower lobe, but no bronchophony or egophony. Musculoskeletal and cutaneous exams are unremarkable. Chest radiographs show a patchy nodular infiltrate in the left lower lobe. Blood, sputum, and urine cultures are obtained.

Which one of the following antibiotics should be administered?
A. Daptomycin.
B. Ceftriaxone.
C. Vancomycin.
D. Streptomycin.

15. A previously healthy 19-year-old male presents to the emergency room following the sudden onset of sharp right-sided chest pain and shortness of breath. The pain radiates into his neck. He denies cough and hemoptysis. Symptoms occurred while he was watching television. He was able to walk to the emergency room as he only lives 3 blocks away. He is a nonsmoker.

On physical examination temperature is 37.3°C, respiratory rate is 20 breaths/min, heart rate is 104 beats/min, and blood pressure is 122/79 mm Hg. Room air oxygen saturation measured by pulse oximetry is 93%. The patient is in no distress. The trachea is midline. Percussion of the chest shows an area of hyperresonance over the anterior upper right thorax. Breath sounds also appear diminished in this region. No crepitation can be appreciated with palpation of the thorax and supraclavicular fossae. Chest radiographs show an approximately 3.2 cm apical right pneumothorax.

Which one of the following is the most appropriate management?

A. Repeat the chest radiographs in 6 hours and, if no change, discharge to home with follow-up in one day.
B. Insert a 12 Fr catheter attached to a water seal device followed by admission to the hospital.
C. Insert a 28 Fr chest tube attached to a water seal device followed by admission to the hospital.
D. Schedule video-assisted thorascopic surgery with bullectomy within the next 24 hours.

16. A 43-year-old female with idiopathic pulmonary arterial hypertension is experiencing worsening shortness of breath upon exertion (New York Heart Association Class IV) despite treatment with bosentan and continuous intravenous epoprostenol. Her most recent right heart catheterization revealed the following hemodynamic parameters: cardiac index 1.8 L/min/m^2, right atrial pressure of 21 mm Hg, and a mean pulmonary artery pressure of 62 mm Hg. She is interested in bilateral lung transplantation.

Which one of the following would be considered an absolute contraindication to lung transplantation?

A. Symptomatic osteoporosis.
B. Kyphoscoliosis.
C. Creatinine clearance of 46 mg/ml/min.
D. History of treated *Mycobacterium tuberculosis* infection.

17. A 39-year-old male presents with worsening shortness of breath, fever, weakness, and skin rash. He has a history of asthma and allergic rhinitis diagnosed approximately 10 years ago. He is a nonsmoker. Current medications include mometasone dry powdered inhaler 220 mcg once daily, levalbuterol metered dose inhaler 2 puffs every 6 hours as needed, and fexofenadine 180 mg once daily.

On physical examination temperature is 38.1°C, heart rate is 84 beats/min, blood pressure is 152/90 mm Hg, and respiratory rate is 20 breaths/min. He does not appear to be in any distress. Cardiac exam reveals a normal S1 and S2. Lung sounds are clear bilaterally. There is no digital clubbing. Cutaneous examination reveals multiple raised purpura involving all extremities. Mild adenopathy is appreciated in the anterior cervical axillary and inguinal regions. There is mild atrophy of the thenar eminences. Left ankle dorsiflexion is diminished.

Laboratory data includes a Westergren erythrocyte sedimentation rate of 102 mm/hr, leukocyte count of 13,000/cu mm with 50% eosinophils, 40% segmented neutrophils, and 10% lymphocytes. Hemoglobin is 12.1 g/dL with an MCV of 94 fL, creatinine is 1.9 mg/dL, and serum IgE is 1,100 IU/mL. ANCA indirect immunofluorescence assay is performed and shows a staining pattern limited to the perinuclear region. Chest radiographs show vague bilateral pulmonary infiltrates. There is a small right pleural effusion.

Which one of the following treatments will be most beneficial?
A. Prednisone.
B. Plasma exchange.
C. Cyclophosphamide and plasma exchange.
D. Intravenous immunoglobulin.

18. A 19-year-old female is undergoing evaluation for chronic back pain. It is localized to the upper thoracic spine. The pain has been present for several years and is gradually getting worse. She has no other complaints. On physical examination there is asymmetry noted with the forward bend test. Posteroanterior and lateral view radiographs of the spine show a Cobb angle of 20°.

Which one of the following about this patient's condition is true?
A. Pulmonary function testing will be normal.
B. Pulmonary function testing will show a reduced total lung capacity.
C. There will be evidence of hypoventilation during rapid eye movement sleep.
D. There will be evidence of chronic hypercapnic respiratory failure with the daytime arterial PCO_2 > 45 mm Hg.

19. Which one of the following statements about chronic eosinophilic pneumonia is true?
A. The chest radiographic findings of dense, extensive, bilateral, peripheral infiltrates are present in the majority of patients at the time of presentation.
B. Coexistent asthma is common.
C. Definitive diagnosis requires a lung biopsy.
D. The majority of patients will require lifelong treatment with glucocorticoids.

20. A 52-year-old male was diagnosed with acquired immune deficiency syndrome approximately 12 years ago after presenting with a wasting syndrome. His course has been complicated by pneumonia due to *Pneumocystis jirovecii*. He is currently receiving antiretroviral therapy with efavirenz, tenofovir, and emtricitabine. Three months ago he developed worsening shortness of breath and mild hemoptysis. Chest radiographs show a density in the left upper lobe. Computed tomography scanning of the chest is performed. A representative image is shown in figure 20-A. Percutaneous core biopsy of the lesion is performed. A representative image is shown in figure 20-B. The patient's most recent CD4 lymphocyte count is 800/cu mm. The plasma viral load is undetectable.

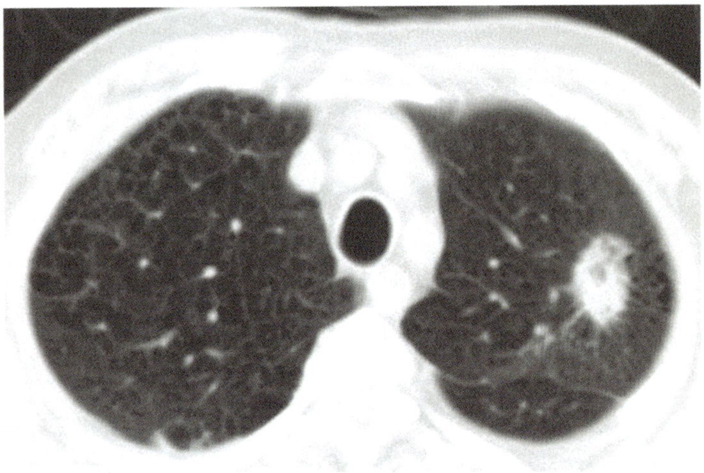

Figure 20-A

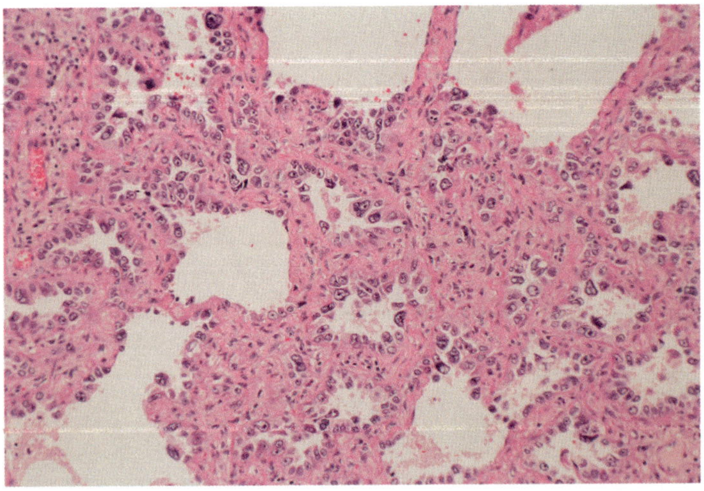

Figure 20-B

Which one of the following statements about this condition is true?
A. The median survival is less than that of age-matched patients not infected with the human immunodeficiency virus.
B. The patient is likely a current or former cigarette smoker.
C. Herpes simplex virus-8 plays a role in the pathogenesis of this condition.
D. The incidence of this condition has decreased in the era of antiretroviral therapy.

21. A 24-year-old female with a history of asthma is transported to the emergency room by an ambulance. She was in her usual state of health until earlier today. She is a teacher at a local elementary school. Shortly after arriving at the school, she began having shortness of breath, cough, and wheezing. She thought her symptoms were triggered by a strong odor in her classroom. A colleague mentioned to her that the school had undergone an industrial cleaning the night before. Her symptoms did not resolve with a total of 4 inhalations of her albuterol rescue inhaler. Emergency medical services were contacted, and the patient was brought to the emergency room.

On physical examination the patient is anxious and in respiratory distress. She is having difficulty speaking in complete sentences. While clutching her upper chest, she states she is "choking." The sternocleidomastoid, trapezius, scalene, and pectoralis muscles are being used to assist with respiration. Respiratory rate is approximately 30 breaths/min, heart rate is 110 beats/min, and blood pressure is 160/95 mm Hg. Pulsus paradoxus is not present. While the patient is receiving continuous albuterol via a nebulizer, her chest is auscultated. There is a high-pitch inspiratory hiss best heard anteriorly. Breath sounds are otherwise diminished bilaterally. As endotracheal intubation is contemplated, the patient begins to dramatically improve.

Which one of the following should be performed next?
A. Rapid sequence intubation using fentanyl, etomidate, and succinylcholine.
B. Provide reassurance and supportive care.
C. Administer methylprednisolone 125 mg intravenously.
D. Administer magnesium sulfate 2 g intravenously.

22. A 67-year-old female is interested in assistance with smoking cessation. She has smoked 2 packs of cigarettes a day for approximately 30 years. She has never before tried to quit. Past medical history includes hypertension, 3-vessel coronary artery disease with stable angina, and epilepsy.

What pharmacological therapy should be recommended?
A. Nicotine transdermal patch.
B. Nicotine transdermal patch with bupropion SR.
C. Bupropion SR.
D. None; pharmacologic therapy is contraindicated with her medical problems.

23. A 69-year-old male presents to the emergency room with complaints of pain and redness involving the right calf. He first noticed the symptoms approximately 72 hours ago. He doesn't recall any trauma to his leg. Symptoms have not improved with use of an over-the-counter nonsteroidal anti-inflammatory medication. Past medical history includes diabetes mellitus, hypertension, and gout. He recently retired from his job as a florist after 40 years. The only recent travel history was a car trip to see his daughter out of state.

On physical examination the patient is afebrile. Blood pressure is 130/84 mm Hg, heart rate is 95 beats/min, and respiratory rate is 18 breaths/min. Auscultation of the heart and lungs is unremarkable. Examination of the right lower extremity reveals mild pitting edema around the ankle. The posterior calf is warm, erythematous, and tender to touch. The right calf is 3 cm larger than the left when measured 10 cm below the tibial tuberosity. Pain is not precipitated with flexion of the knee and dorsiflexion of the ankle.

The most likely diagnosis is:
A. Cellulitis.
B. Deep venous thrombosis.
C. Popliteal cyst.
D. Muscle strain.

24. A 52-year-old female undergoes preemployment chest radiographs that demonstrate a right middle lobe nodule. This lesion was not present on a prior study done 2 years ago when the patient had an acute respiratory illness. She currently feels well and denies any shortness of breath, cough, hemoptysis, or wheezing. A review of systems is negative for fever, weight loss, muscle wasting, skin rash, and diarrhea. She has an approximately 15-pack-year history of smoking cigarettes. Physical examination is normal. Complete blood count and complete metabolic panel are normal. Computed tomography scanning of the chest is performed. A representative image is shown in figure 24-A. Following this, a percutaneous core biopsy is performed. A representative image is shown in figure 24-B.

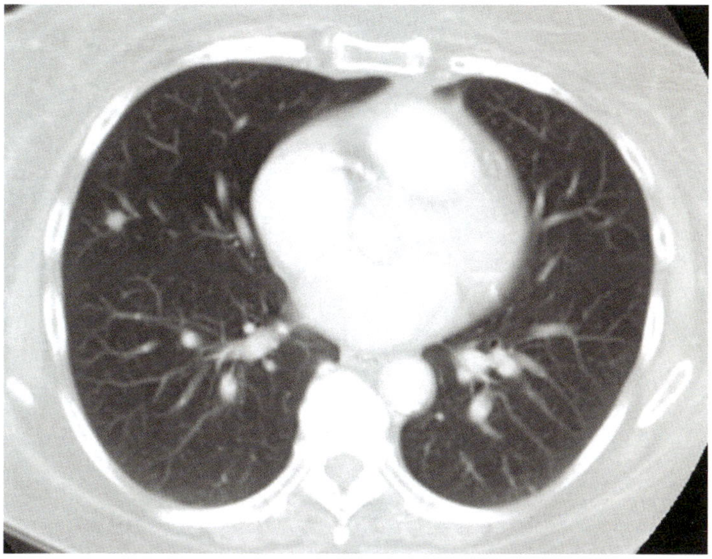

Figure 24-A

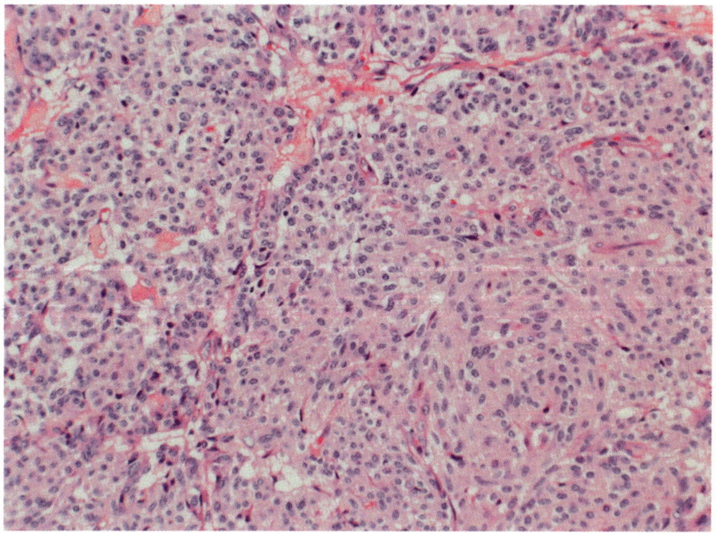

Figure 24-B

Which one of the following should be performed next?

A. Somatostatin receptor scintigraphy.
B. Thoracotomy with right upper lobectomy and mediastinal lymph node dissection.
C. Measurement of 24-hour urinary level of 5-hydroxyindoleacetic acid.
D. Measurement of serum chromogranin A.

25. A 28-year-old female, primigravida, in the 34th week of pregnancy, is admitted to the obstetrical unit with preterm labor contractions. Past medical history includes insulin-dependent diabetes mellitus. At the time of admission she is treated with intravenous terbutaline. Approximately 24 hours later, the patient develops orthopnea and dyspnea with exertion. On physical examination temperature is 36.7°C, heart rate is 113 beats/min, respiratory rate is 28 breaths/min, and blood pressure is 129/84 mm Hg. With the patient at a 45° incline, jugular venous distention cannot be appreciated. Cardiac examination reveals a normal S1 and S2 with a medium-pitched, early systolic murmur best heard at the 2nd left interspace. Auscultation of the lungs is notable for bibasilar inspiratory crackles. A single view portable chest radiograph shows haziness involving the perihilar regions bilaterally, prominent septal lines, and patchy bilateral lung densities. Brain natriuretic peptide is 102 pg/ml. Hemoglobin, leukocyte count, and platelet count are normal.

Which one of the following statements about this condition is true?

A. Survivors may require cardiac transplantation.
B. Mechanical ventilation is necessary in the majority of patients.
C. It is the leading cause of maternal death.
D. With appropriate treatment the syndrome will usually resolve within 24 hours.

26. Which one of the following statements about nonspecific interstitial pneumonia is true?

A. Pulmonary function testing usually shows a pattern of obstruction with a markedly reduced diffusion capacity.
B. A causal association with cigarette smoking has been established.
C. Has a better prognosis than usual interstitial pneumonitis.
D. Computed tomography scanning of the chest typically shows diffuse ground glass opacities with honeycombing.

27. A 62-year-old male is referred for evaluation of a right pleural effusion. About 2 weeks ago he developed a new onset illness characterized by low-grade fever, pleuritic chest pain, and a nonproductive cough. Chest radiographs performed at that time showed a small right pleural effusion. He was treated for presumed community-acquired pneumonia with a course of azithromycin. Symptoms did not improve, and repeat chest radiographs showed a persistent effusion. Past medical history includes alcoholism. As a young man he served in the military and was briefly deployed on a naval warship. Following this, he was a long-distance truck driver until his retirement about 8 months ago. He is twice divorced and estranged from his children.

On physical examination temperature is 36.8°C, respiratory rate is 16 breaths/min, heart rate is 72 beats/min, and blood pressure is 142/83 mm Hg. Inspection of the thorax is unremarkable. Skodaic resonance is present above the posterior right chest at the 8th intercostal space. Vocal fremitus and vocal sounds are absent at the right base. A diagnostic thoracentesis is performed with removal of approximately 200 ml of straw-colored fluid. The fluid has 5,000 nucleated cells/microL with a differential of 90% lymphocytes, 8% neutrophils, 1% mesothelial cells, and 1% eosinophils. Protein is 5.2 g/dL, glucose is 70 mg/dL, and pH is 7.30. Cytologic analysis does not show any malignant cells.

Which one of the following should be performed next?
A. Decortication.
B. Observation.
C. Treatment with isoniazid, rifampin, pyrazinamide, and ethambutol.
D. Ventilation/perfusion scan.

28. A 57-year-old nonsmoking male presents with a 1-year history of dry cough, throat clearing, and intermittent hoarseness. Past medical history is notable for essential hypertension. Current medications are lisinopril 10 mg orally once a day and an over-the-counter antihistamine as needed. He works as a receptionist at a financial investment firm. He frequently visits his sister who has 2 indoor cats.

On physical examination the conjunctivae do not appear injected. Nasal mucosa is moist without erythema. Direct laryngoscopy shows edematous changes to the true and false vocal cords. Auscultation of the thorax demonstrates bronchial breath sounds over the manubrium, bronchovesicular breath sounds along the second and third intercostal spaces, and vesicular breath sounds at the lung periphery bilaterally. Diagnostic evaluation includes a bronchoprovocation test that shows a 20% decrease in the FEV_1 after a total methacholine concentration of 16 mg/ml. Skin testing to grass, tree, weed pollens, and cat dander are negative. Posteroanterior and lateral view chest radiographs are shown in figures 28-A and 28-B respectively.

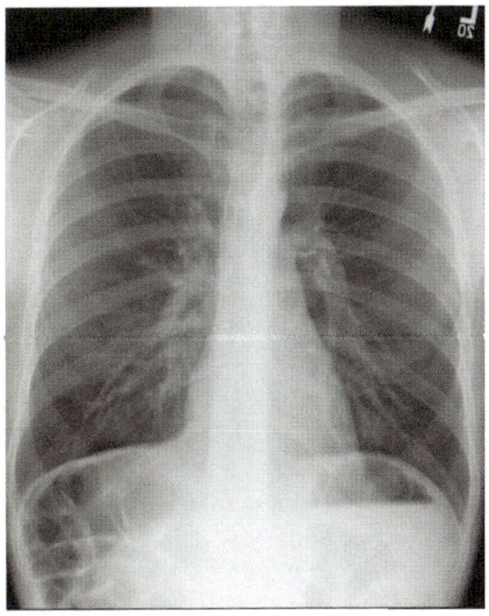

Figure 28-A

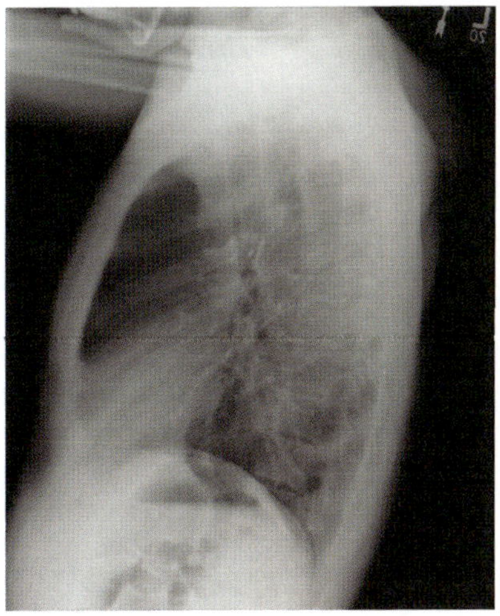

Figure 28-B

Which one of the following interventions should be performed next?
A. Refer to speech therapy for breathing and voice exercises.
B. Begin a long-acting beta agonist.
C. Discontinue lisinopril.
D. Perform behavior modification and dietary changes.

29. A community hospital is starting a comprehensive pulmonary rehabilitation program for patients with chronic obstructive lung disease. Which one of the following should not be a mandatory component of the curriculum?
A. Inspiratory muscle training.
B. High-intensity lower extremity exercises.
C. Unsupported endurance training of the upper extremities.
D. Strength training added to endurance training.

30. A 66-year-old male is admitted to the hospital with gastrointestinal bleeding. He was in his usual state of health until 2 days ago when he developed left lower quadrant cramping abdominal pain followed by multiple loose stools. He noticed with each bowel movement the presence of bright red blood. This morning he decided to seek medical attention when he felt dizzy and had palpitations getting out of bed. He has no prior history of gastrointestinal bleeding. Past medical history is positive for paroxysmal atrial fibrillation treated with sotalol and warfarin.

On physical examination temperature is 37.2°C, heart rate is 120 beats/min, respiratory rate of 17 breaths/min, and supine blood pressure is 95/60 mm Hg. Examination of the neck reveals no jugular venous distension. Abdominal exam shows some tenderness in the left lower quadrant and epigastric areas, but no guarding or rebound is present. Digital rectal examination reveals no hemorrhoids. Laboratory data shows a hemoglobin of 8.5 g/dL, platelet count of 250,000/cu mm, partial thromboplastin time of 35 seconds, and a protime of 20 seconds.

Resuscitation efforts are started in the emergency room with the administration of intravenous normal saline bolus, transfusions of fresh frozen plasma, and packed red blood cells. Approximately 30 minutes later, the patient begins to experience breathing problems. Repeat examination now shows a temperature of 38.2°C, heart rate of 125 beats/min, respiratory rate of 28 breaths/min, and blood pressure of 100/60 mm Hg. Pulse oximetry performed on room air shows an oxygen saturation of 85%. He is in moderate respiratory distress and using accessory muscles to assist with breathing. Auscultation of the lungs reveals late inspiratory crackles bilaterally. A stat portable anteroposterior chest radiograph shows bilateral pulmonary densities. Because of worsening respiratory distress, the patient undergoes emergent oral endotracheal intubation with initiation of mechanical ventilation.

Which one of the follow statements about this condition is false?

A. It may have been precipitated by leukocyte antibodies in the fresh frozen plasma.
B. It may have been precipitated by biologically active cytokines in the packed red blood cells.
C. The mortality rate is similar to other causes of acute lung injury.
D. With appropriate supportive care, the syndrome will likely resolve within 3 days.

31. A 72-year-old female complains of progressive shortness of breath, cough, chest pain, and fatigue for the past 2 months. She denies weight loss, skin rash, or muscle pain. She is a lifelong nonsmoker. Past medical history includes recurrent cystitis, hypertension, and osteoporosis. Current medications are hydrochlorothiazide, calcium with vitamin D, alendronate, aspirin, and nitrofurantoin.

On physical examination vital signs are stable. Curved kyphosis is noted upon inspection of the chest. Excursion of the posterior chest is normal. Auscultation of the lungs demonstrates early inspiratory fine crackles bilaterally. No wheezes are appreciated. Dermatologic exam is unremarkable. Pulmonary function test shows a total lung capacity of 68% of predicted, FVC of 71% of predicted, FEV_1 of 75% of predicted. Diffusion capacity is 69% of predicted. Oxygen saturation on room air measured by pulse oximeter at rest is 95% and decreases to 90% with ambulation. Serum ALT is 80 U/L, AST is 74 U/L, and ANA is 1:40. Posteroanterior and lateral view chest radiographs show diffuse interstitial changes bilaterally. Computed tomography scanning of the chest is performed. A representative image is shown in figure 31-A.

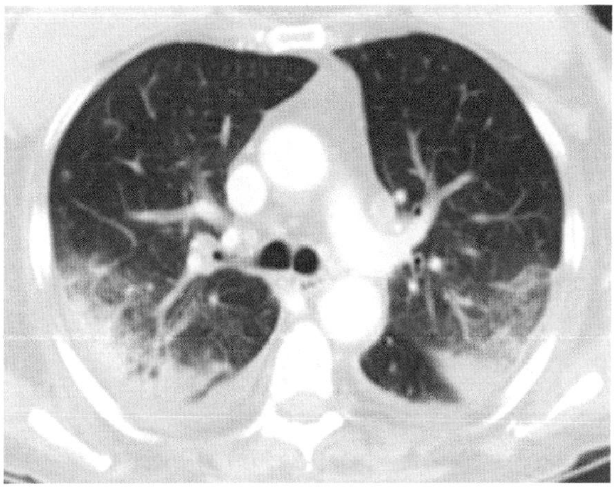

Figure 31-A

Which one of the following statements about the chronic form of this condition is false?

A. It is the result of a hypersensitivity pneumonitis.
B. Digital clubbing is rare.
C. Peripheral eosinophilia may be present.
D. Pleural effusions are uncommon.

32. A previously healthy 52-year-old female presents to the emergency room with worsening shortness of breath. She was in her usual state of health until approximately 3 weeks ago when she developed a flu-like illness characterized by headache, muscle soreness, sore throat, cough, shortness of breath, and low-grade fever. She is married with 3 healthy children. She is a lifelong nonsmoker. She denies owning pets and has no recent travel history. She has no known risk factors for infection with the human immunodeficiency virus.

On physical examination temperature is 38.1°C, respiratory rate is 28 breaths/min, heart rate is 111 beats/min, and blood pressure is 160/89 mm Hg. She is in mild distress but not using accessory muscles to assist with respirations. Inspection, percussion, and vibratory palpation of the thorax are unremarkable. Auscultation of the lungs is notable for early inspiratory fine crackles at the bases that do not clear with coughing. No cardiac murmurs or gallops are present. There is no evidence of skin rash, synovitis, or muscle weakness.

A portable anteroposterior chest radiograph is shown in figure 32-A. Leukocyte count is 11,000/cu mm with 65% segmented neutrophils, 5% band forms, 28% lymphocytes, 2% eosinophils. Hemoglobin

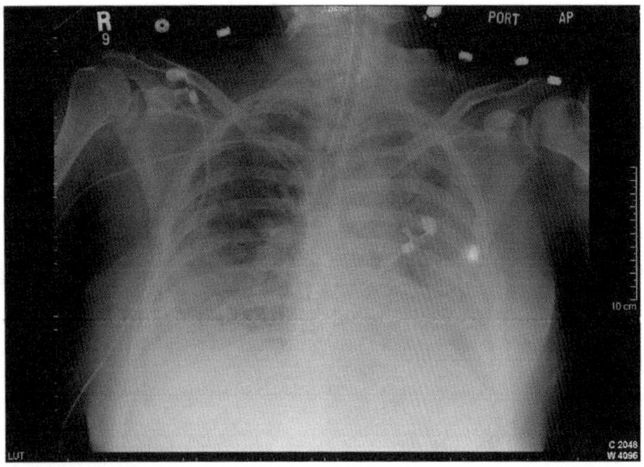

Figure 32-A

is 14 g/dL, platelet count is 300,000/cu mm, brain natriuretic peptide is 160 pg/mL, creatinine is 0.8 mg/dL, and creatinine kinase is 48 U/L. A urine toxicology screen is negative. Blood cultures and a urinary Legionella antigen are obtained in the emergency room. The patient is started on intravenous ceftriaxone and azithromycin and admitted to the intensive care unit.

Over the next 24 hours the patient becomes progressively more hypoxic and requires endotracheal intubation and mechanical ventilation. Bronchoscopy with bronchoalveolar lavage is performed in the medial segment of the right middle lobe with a return of clear fluid with a predominance of neutrophils. Bacterial gram stain does not show any organisms. Smears for acid-fast bacilli and fungi are negative.

Which one of the following about this condition is true?

A. There will be a rapid improvement following the administration of intravenous glucocorticoids.
B. Relapse is uncommon.
C. With supportive care the majority will survive.
D. Lung biopsy will show features of diffuse alveolar damage.

33. A 64-year-old male is evaluated for a 6-week history of a cough productive of blood-streaked sputum, shortness of breath, and a 10-pound weight loss. He sought medical attention at a local walk-in clinic where chest radiographs showed an ill-defined density in the right lower lobe. His symptoms and the radiographic findings did not improve with a course of moxifloxacin for presumed community-acquired pneumonia. Habits include smoking 1 pack of cigarettes and consuming a 6-pack of beer daily.

On physical examination temperature is 36.5°C, pulse rate is 90/min, respiratory rate is14/min, and blood pressure is 118/75 mmHg. Lung auscultation reveals right lower lobe mid-to-late inspiratory crackles. No cardiac murmurs, gallops, or friction rubs are present. Examination of the oral cavity reveals that the right lower first bicuspid and the upper left incisor teeth are absent. There is no peripheral edema or hepatosplenomegaly. Computer tomography scanning of his chest following the administration of intravenous contrast shows an area of consolidation at the periphery of the right lower lobe. Hilar and mediastinal adenopathy are not appreciated. There are no pleural effusions.

Because of the concern for bronchogenic carcinoma, the patient undergoes an ultrasound-guided percutaneous core biopsy of the lesion. A representative image is shown in figure 33-A. Tissue gram stain is shown in figure 33-B. No organisms are appreciated after the tissue is prepared using the Kinyoun procedure.

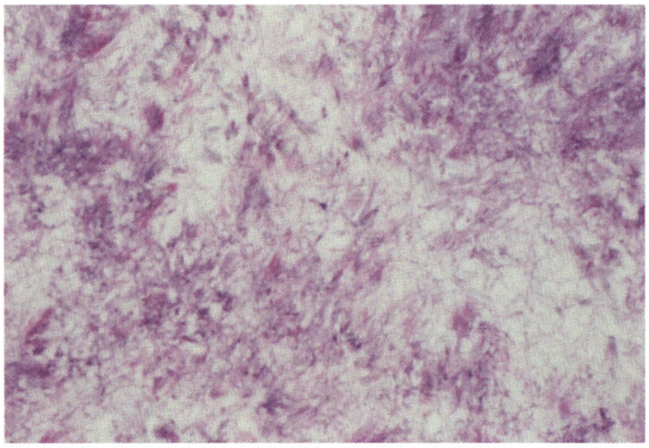

Figure 33-A

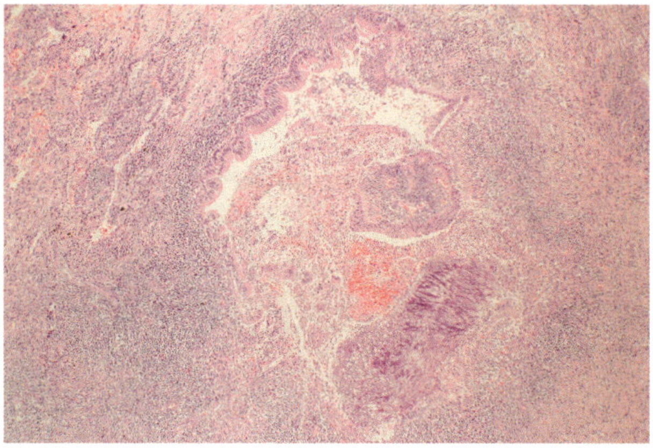

Figure 33-B

The diagnosis is:

A. Adenocarcinoma of lung primary, with a papillary growth pattern.
B. Actinomycosis.
C. Tuberculosis.
D. Nocardiosis.

34. A 38-year-old female is referred for evaluation of persistent, moderate-sized bilateral pleural effusions. She originally presented to her primary care physician approximately 4 weeks ago with shortness of breath and lower extremity edema. Diagnostic studies at that time included chest radiographs that showed moderate-size pleural effusions and a normal-size cardiac silhouette. Electrocardiogram revealed normal sinus rhythm. Brain natriuretic peptide was 150 pg/mL, serum creatinine was 0.8 mg/dL, and albumin was 3.7 g/dL. Urinalysis did not show any red blood cell casts or proteinuria. The patient is otherwise healthy except for intermittent episodes of sinusitis and bronchitis requiring antimicrobial therapy 2 to 3 times each year. She denies any known tuberculosis exposure. She works at a local veterinary clinic primarily doing clerical work. Family history is unremarkable. She is a lifelong nonsmoker.

On physical examination she is afebrile. The respiratory rate is 16 breaths/min. Non-pitting edema can be appreciated around the eyelids, fingertips, and ankles. The nails on both hands appear slightly thickened and an overcurvature is present. Auscultation of the heart reveals a normal S1 and S2 without any gallops. Lung sounds are diminished at the bases. There is also dullness to percussion over these regions. Egophony and bronchophony are not present.

A diagnostic thoracentesis is performed. Pleural fluid analysis is expected to show which one of the following?

A. Greater than 100,000 nucleated cells/microL with a predominance of neutrophils, pH < 7.20, protein > 5 g/dL, and an LDH > 1,000 U/L.
B. Total nucleated cells > 5,000/microL with a predominance of neutrophils. Rare phagocytic leukocytes with inclusion bodies are present. The glucose is less than 60 mg/dL, pH < 7.30.
C. Blood-tinged fluid with pronounced eosinophilia. Protein is 4.5 g/dL and LDH is 300 U/L.
D. Straw-colored fluid with less than 1,000/microL cells with a predominance of lymphocytes. Total protein concentration is 3.6 g/dL and the LDH is 150 U/L.

35. Recurrence of the primary disease after lung transplantation is most likely to occur with which one of the following?

A. Sarcoidosis.
B. Pulmonary alveolar proteinosis.
C. Bronchoalveolar cell carcinoma.
D. Pulmonary Langerhans'- cell histiocytosis.

36. A 61-year-old female presents with several weeks of fever, poor appetite, 11-pound weight loss, and fatigue. A review of systems is positive for runny nose with occasional blood-streaked discharge, dry cough, shortness of breath with exertion, and a rash on the lower extremities. Past medical history is positive for cataracts, obstructive sleep apnea being treated with continuous positive airway pressure, and a prior appendectomy. Her only medication is an over-the-counter multivitamin with minerals.

On physical examination temperature is 38.2°C, heart rate is 84 beats/min, blood pressure is 171/90 mm Hg, and respiratory rate is 16 breaths/min. The patient is in no distress. Conjunctivae appear normal. The dorsum of the nose is sunken, and there is crusting of the nares bilaterally. Cardiopulmonary and abdominal examinations are unremarkable. The skin on the lower extremities has a mesh-like appearance with numerous blue-purple streaks present.

Diagnostic studies include a Westergren erythrocyte sedimentation rate of 104 mm/hr, leukocyte count of 12,000/cu mm with a normal differential, hemoglobin of 10.8 g/dL with a MCV of 87 fL, BUN of 28 mg/dL, creatinine of 1.9 mg/dL, and a urinalysis that reveals numerous dysmorphic red blood cells. Indirect immunofluorescent assay for ANCA is positive. The enzyme-linked immunoassay shows antibodies against proteinase-3. Chest radiographs show discreet pulmonary nodules with right hilar adenopathy.

Which one of the following is the most common tracheobronchial abnormality that occurs with this condition?

A. Subglottic stenosis.
B. Bronchial stenosis.
C. Tracheomalacia.
D. Bronchomalacia.

37. A previously healthy male presents with new onset shortness of breath. His posteroanterior chest radiograph is shown in figure 37-A. Pulmonary function testing is performed.

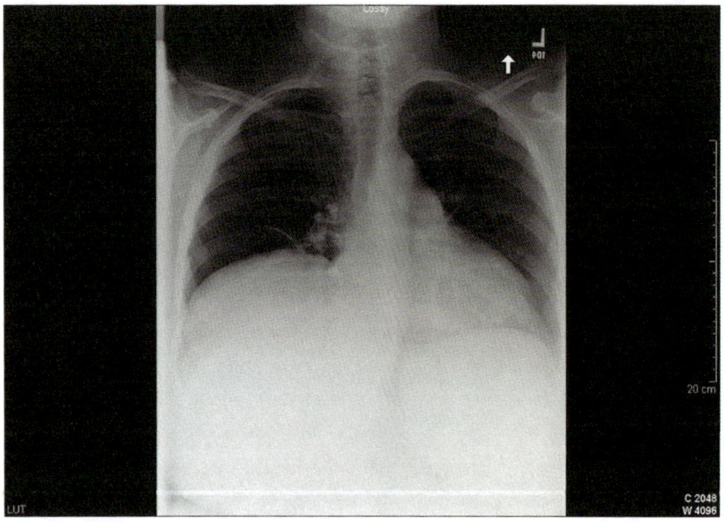

Figure 37-A

Which one of the following will be normal?

A. Vital capacity in the sitting position.
B. Vital capacity in the supine position.
C. Maximal inspiratory pressure.
D. Maximal expiratory pressure.

38. A 54-year-old female is evaluated for a 2-year history of a recurrent illness characterized by chest tightness, shortness of breath, nonproductive cough, and fever. Prior evaluations have been nondiagnostic. The most recent episode started 24 hours after entertaining some friends at her home. Activities included outdoor barbeque and swimming. Past medical history is positive for bronchitis.

She is on no prescription medications. She works part time at a tanning salon. A review of symptoms is positive for a 5-pound weight loss over the last 3 months.

On physical examination the temperature is 38.1°C, heart rate is 86 beats/min, blood pressure is 141/86 mm Hg, and respiratory rate is 20 breaths/min. Cardiac examination demonstrates a normal S1 and S2. Auscultation of the lungs reveals fine inspiratory crackles involving the lower lobes. Digital clubbing is absent. Musculoskeletal and cutaneous examinations are also unremarkable. Postbronchodilator spirometry shows an FEV_1 of 1.92 L (71% of predicted), FVC of 2.62 L (73% of predicted), and an FEV_1/FVC of 73%. Chest radiographs show subtle micronodular opacities in the middle to upper lung zones. High-resolution computed tomography scanning confirms diffuse micronodules and nonspecific ground glass opacities.

Which one of the following about this case is most likely to be true?

A. The individual is most likely a nonsmoker.
B. Serial exhaled nitric oxide levels are useful to monitor disease course.
C. Analysis of bronchoalveolar lavage fluid lymphocyte subsets will show a CD4/CD8 ratio > 1.0.
D. A diagnosis can be made if serum precipitating IgG antibodies are positive.

39. A 58-year-old male with a history of fibrocavitary sarcoidosis presents with hemoptysis for the past 3 weeks. He is expectorating several milliliters of bright red blood daily. The volume of blood has gradually increased. He has chronic dyspnea with all exertion at baseline. He has no other chronic medical conditions and is on no current medications. Physical examination is unremarkable. Chest radiographs show a mass within a cavity in the left upper lobe. Computed tomography scanning of the chest is performed. A representative image is shown in figure 39-A. Pulmonary function testing shows a postbronchodilator FEV_1 of 1.2 liters and a diffusion capacity of 36% of predicted. The VO_2 maximum obtained during a treadmill cardiopulmonary exercise test is 9 ml/kg/min.

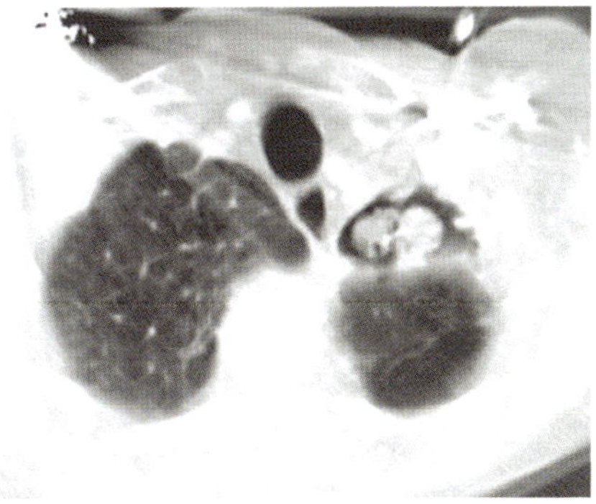

Figure 39-A

Which one of the following would be the optimal treatment strategy for this patient?
A. Right upper lobectomy.
B. Endobronchial catheter placement with installation of Amphotericin B into the cavity.
C. Oral itraconazole 200 mg twice daily.
D. Bronchial artery embolization.

40. Which one of the following is the most common side effect of inhaled glucocorticoids?
A. Oropharyngeal candidiasis.
B. Perioral dermatitis.
C. Dysphonia.
D. Pharyngitis.

41. The most common cause of death in patients with chronic obstructive pulmonary disease is:
A. Bronchogenic carcinoma.
B. Bacterial pneumonia.
C. Pulmonary embolism.
D. Ischemic heart disease.

42. Which one of the following is the most common chest radiographic abnormality in a patient with an acute pulmonary embolism?
A. Focal area of avascularity.
B. Pleural effusion.
C. Prominence of the central pulmonary artery.
D. Pleural-based wedge-shaped density.

43. A 64-year-old male is found to have a new left lung nodule, illustrated in figure 43-A. Positron emission tomography is performed following the administration of (18) F-2-deoxy-2-fluor-D-glucose. A representative image is shown in figure 43-B. A percutaneous core biopsy is shown in figure 43-C.

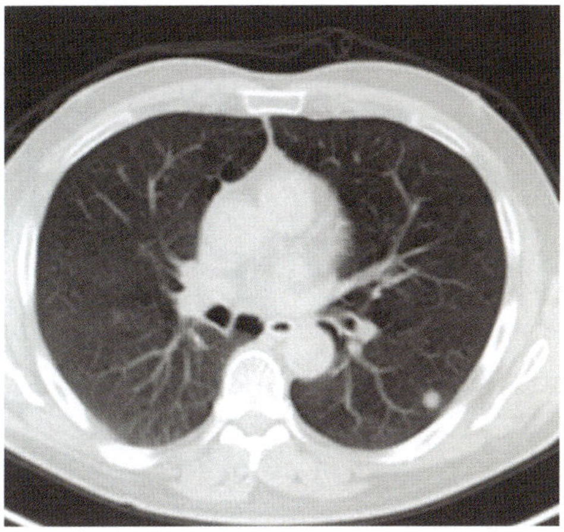

Figure 43-A

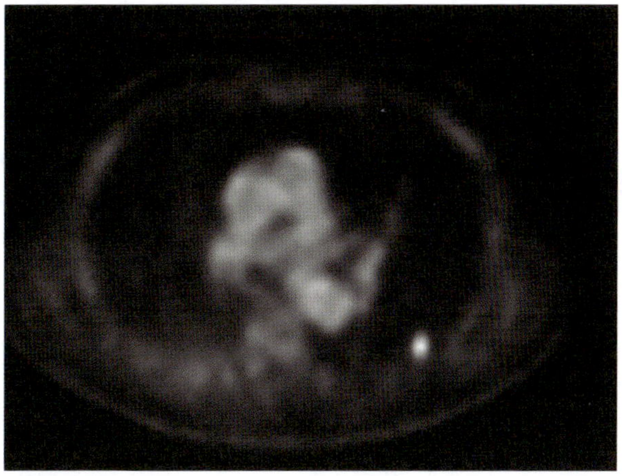

Figure 43-B

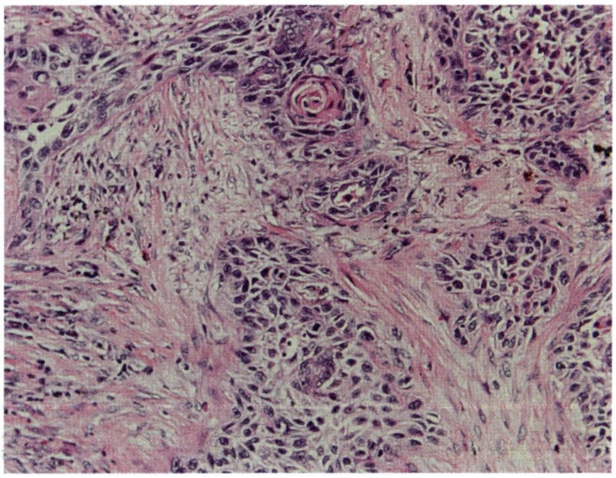

Figure 43-C

Which one of the following symptoms is the patient most likely experiencing?

A. Digital clubbing and pain in the lower extremities bilaterally.
B. Nausea, vomiting, anorexia, constipation, lethargy, and dehydration.
C. Cutaneous flushing, diarrhea, cough, and wheezing.
D. Ring scotomas, night blindness, and photosensitivity.

44. A 26-year-old female with acquired immunodeficiency syndrome presents with night sweats, fatigue, anorexia, cachexia, fever, and cough. CD4 lymphocyte count is 390/cc mm. Chest radiographs show diffuse parenchymal densities, as illustrated in figure 44-A. Computed tomography scanning of the chest is performed. A representative image is shown in figure 44-B. A tuberculin skin test shows no induration. Three sputa are induced using hypertonic saline. All 3 samples are smear-positive for acid-fast bacilli. A nucleic acid amplification assay is positive for *Mycobacterium tuberculosis* DNA. Current medications include darunavir-ritonavir and tenofovir-emtricitabine.

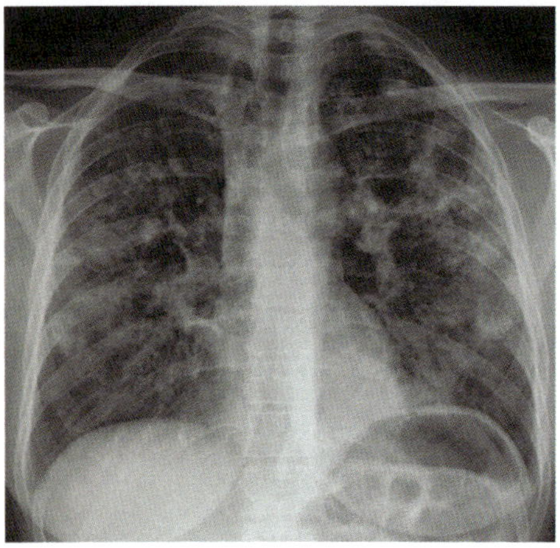

Figure 44-A

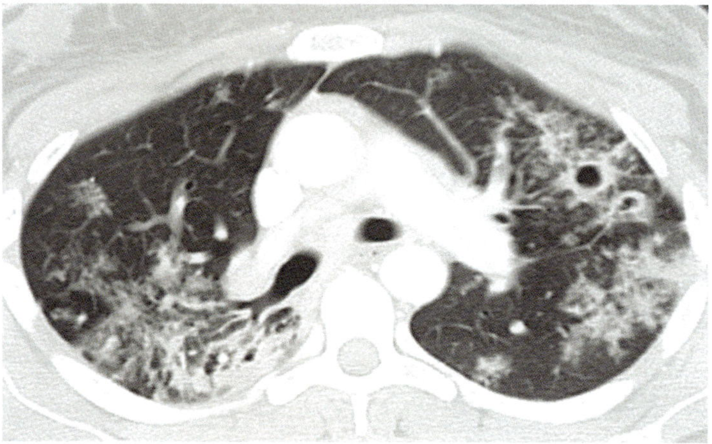

Figure 44-B

Which one of the following drug regimens should not be used for treatment?

A. Isoniazid, rifabutine, pyrazinamide, and ethambutol daily for 8 weeks followed by isoniazid and rifabutine daily for 18 weeks.

B. Isoniazid, rifabutine, pyrazinamide, and ethambutol daily for 8 weeks followed by isoniazid and rifabutine 5 days a week for 18 weeks.

C. Isoniazid, rifabutine, pyrazinamide, and ethambutol 3 times weekly for 8 weeks followed by isoniazid and rifabutine 3 times weekly for 18 weeks.

D. Isoniazid, rifabutine, pyrazinamide, and ethambutol daily for 8 weeks followed by isoniazid and rifabutine twice weekly for 18 weeks.

45. A 21-year-old female, gravida 2, para 1, is at 33 weeks of gestation. She presents to the emergency room with chest tightness, shortness of breath, cough, and wheezing. Symptoms started shortly after being exposed to a cat at a baby shower hosted by her mother-in-law. The patient has a history of asthma and allergic rhinitis. Her respiratory conditions have been well controlled during the pregnancy with inhaled fluticasone 44 mcg 2 inhalations twice daily, albuterol 2 inhalations every 6 hours as needed, and loratadine 10 mg orally once a day.

On physical examination the patient appears mildly uncomfortable. Temperature is 37.1°C, and respiratory rate is 28 breaths/min. The alae nasi are not flaring. No jugular venous distention is present. Hyperresonance is noted with percussion of the thorax. Expiration appears prolonged. Auscultation of the lungs reveals continuous wheezes bilaterally. Heart rhythm is regular. The uterus size is consistent with gestational age and fetal heart tones are present. Treatment is initiated with a combination of albuterol and ipratropium delivered via a jet nebulizer and methylprednisolone 40 mg administered intravenously.

Approximately 30 minutes later, the patient is re-examined. Respiratory rate has decreased to 20 breaths/min and auscultation of the lungs reveals only rare end expiratory wheezes. An arterial blood gas obtained on room air shows a pH of 7.40, $PaCO_2$ of 38 mm Hg, and PaO_2 of 92 mm Hg.

Which one of the following should be performed next?

A. Discharge the patient with a prescription for prednisone and have her see her obstetrician tomorrow.
B. Discharge the patient with prescriptions for prednisone and amoxicillin and have her see her obstetrician tomorrow.
C. Admission to the intensive care unit.
D. Admission to the obstetric unit.

46. A 48-year-old male presents with a several-month history of shortness of breath, cough, fever, diminished appetite, and a 10-pound weight loss. He denies chest pain and hemoptysis. He has a 20-pack-year history of smoking cigarettes. Family history is unremarkable. He works as an athletic trainer at a nearby community college. He is sexually active and has unprotected intercourse with his female partner.

On physical examination temperature is 37.3°C, respiratory rate is 18 breaths/min, heart rate is 86 beats/min, and blood pressure is 132/86 mm Hg. There is no digital clubbing. Inspection and palpation of the thorax are unremarkable. Auscultation of the lungs reveals clear breath sounds. There is no evidence of hepatosplenomegaly. Musculoskeletal and cutaneous exams are normal. Pulmonary function test shows a post bronchodilator FEV_1 of 72% of predicted and FEV_1/FVC ratio of 68%. Lung volumes are normal. The diffusion capacity is 69% of predicted. Posteroanterior and lateral view chest radiographs show micronodular infiltrates and cysts with a predilection for the middle and upper lobes bilaterally. High-resolution computed tomography scanning of the chest is performed. Representative images are shown below in figures 46-A and 46-B. Bronchoscopy with bronchoalveolar lavage of the superior segment of the lingual is performed. The fluid shows abundant histiocytes that stain positive for CD1a.

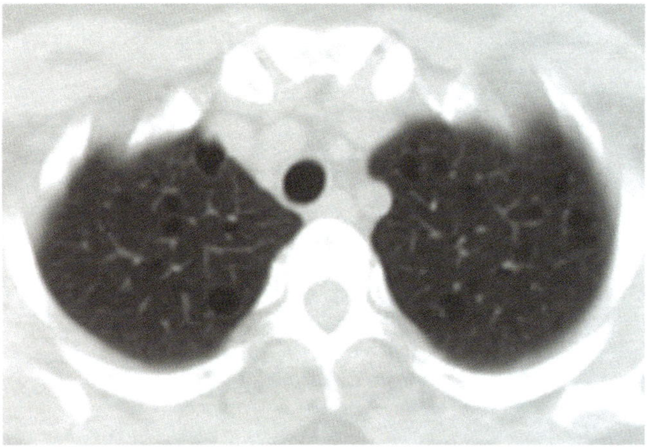

Figure 46-A

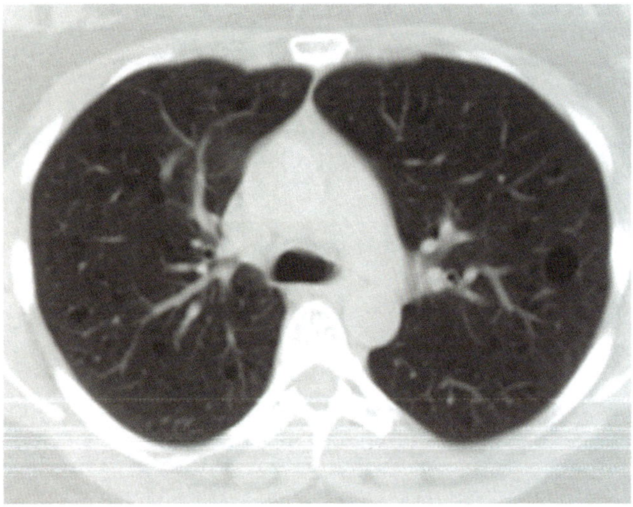

Figure 46-B

All the following statements about this condition are true except:

A. Spontaneous pneumothorax is often the presenting symptom.
B. Bronchoalveolar lavage findings can be diagnostic.
C. Secondary pulmonary hypertension is usually mild and of no clinical significance.
D. The minority of patients will have extrapulmonary manifestations such as cystic bone lesions.

47. A 57-year-old male from Central Illinois presents with a complaint of worsening shortness of breath and a nonproductive cough. A review of systems is positive for a sensation of head fullness, fatigue, and decreased appetite. On physical examination vital signs are stable. Facial plethora and chemosis are present. Venous distention involving the neck, arms, and upper chest is evident. The neck veins do not collapse with inspiration. With extension of his arms above his head he complains of dizziness. Auscultation of the heart reveals an S1 and S2 without any murmur or gallop. The radial pulse does not weaken during inspiration. Computed tomography scanning of the chest with the administration of intravenous contrast is performed. A representative image is shown in figure 47-A.

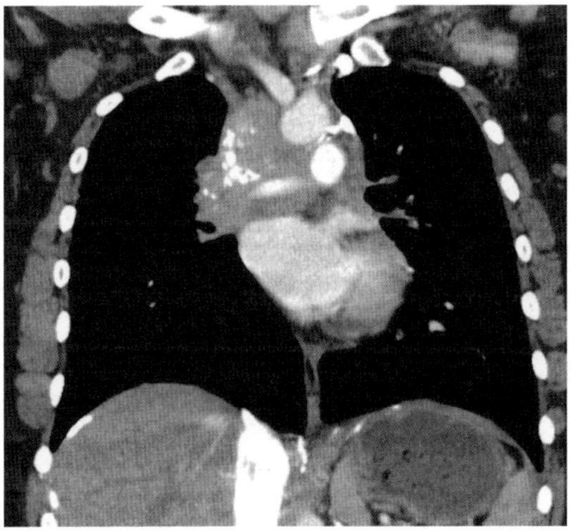

Figure 47-A

Which one of the following should be performed?
A. Administer oral itraconazole 400 mg once daily.
B. Administer prednisone 1 mg/kg orally once daily.
C. Endovascular stent placement.
D. External beam radiation to the mass.

48. A previously healthy 16-year-old male is undergoing evaluation for respiratory complaints. He is on the school indoor ice hockey team. He started to notice symptoms shortly after the season started. He experiences a sensation of chest tightness associated with coughing toward the end of practice. The symptoms initially were quick to resolve with cessation of exercise; however, more recently they have persisted for about an hour. Some of the episodes have been accompanied by wheezing. He denies symptoms of nasal congestion, postnasal drip, and laryngitis.

On physical examination a mild pectus excavatum is present. Heart rhythm is regular with a rate of 74 beats/min. Respiratory rate is 16 breaths/min. With the patient lying supine, there is a short, low-pitched apical murmur that is slightly louder along the sternal border at the left 3rd and 4th intercostal space. The murmur intensifies when he bears down. The lungs are clear to auscultation. There is no digital clubbing.

Which one of the following statements about this condition is false?

A. During the first few minutes of exercise there is an initial bronchoconstriction.
B. During the first few minutes of exercise there is an initial bronchodilation.
C. Peak bronchoconstriction usually occurs within 15 minutes after initiating exercise.
D. Repeated exertion causes less bronchoconstriction.

49. A 20-year-old male with a history of recurrent otitis media, nasal polyposis, and multiple chest infections is undergoing evaluation for infertility. On physical examination vital signs are normal. Precordial palpation shows the point of maximum cardiac impulse to be at the right 5th intercostal space along the midclavicular line. Examination of the abdomen demonstrates an area of tympany in the right upper quadrant. No adventitious sounds are appreciated with auscultation of the lungs. Electrocardiogram shows sinus rhythm with a right axis deviation and low voltage QRS in leads V_4–V_6. Chest radiographs are performed. The posteroanterior view is shown in figure 49-A.

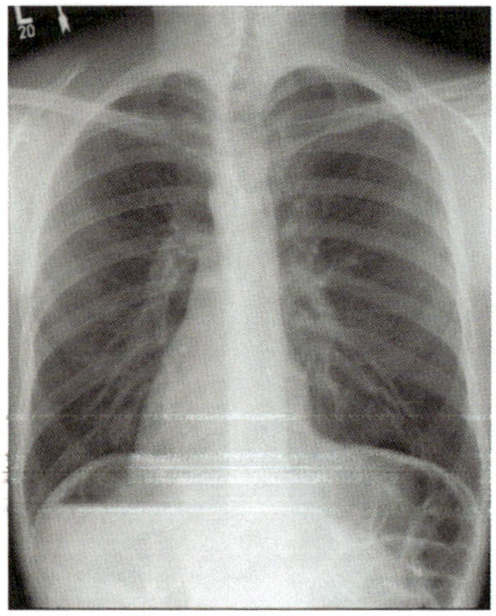

Figure 49-A

Which one of the following statements about this condition is true?

A. A high-resolution computed tomography scan of the chest will reveal traction bronchiectasis.
B. It is an autosomal recessive disease.
C. Circulatory problems lead to a less than normal lifespan.
D. The majority of women are able to successfully conceive and carry a pregnancy to term.

50. A former professional wrestler announces his intention to climb the highest mountain on each continent to raise money for charity. He plans on starting with Mount Kilimanjaro in Africa (peak elevation 5,895 m).

To prevent high altitude pulmonary edema, which one of the following should be administered?
A. Nifedipine.
B. Acetazolamide.
C. Albuterol.
D. Sildenafil.

51. A 42-year-old female complains of new onset shortness of breath, pleurisy, and a cough that is nonproductive. She has classical Hodgkin lymphoma and just completed a 4th cycle of doxorubicin, bleomycin, vinblastine, and dacarbazine. Past medical history is otherwise unremarkable. Family history is positive for early coronary artery disease in her father and one sibling. She denies smoking but admits to having a glass of red wine with dinner every night.

On physical examination vital signs are normal. Oxygen saturation measured by pulse oximetry is 94% on room air. She has diffuse alopecia. Auscultation of the heart does not identify any murmurs or gallops. Lung sounds are positive for mid-to-late fine inspiratory crackles at the bases that do not clear with coughing. Inspection of the abdomen shows a normal contour and no visible masses. The liver edge and spleen tip cannot be felt. The superficial lymph nodes of the neck, axilla, and inguinal regions do not appear enlarged. Computed tomography scanning of the chest is performed. Representative images are shown in figures 51-A and 51-B.

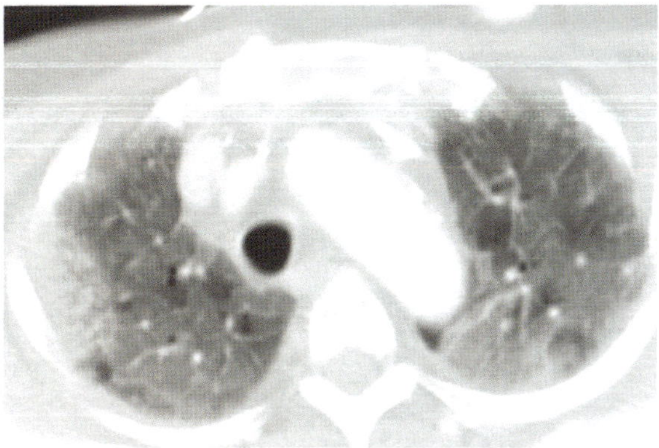

Figure 51-A

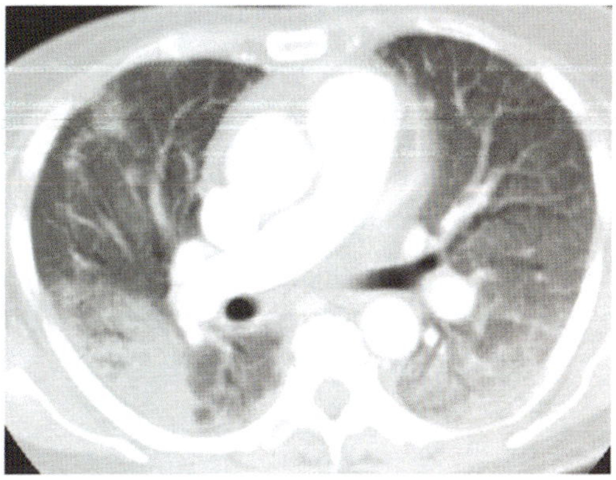

Figure 51-B

Which one of the following is not a risk factor for this condition?
A. Cumulative drug dose.
B. Cigarette smoking.
C. Renal failure.
D. Hepatic failure.

52. A 55-year-old male is evaluated for worsening shortness of breath and cough. The illness started about 2 months ago with fever, fatigue, and anorexia. Progressive shortness of breath and cough soon followed. He was seen in a local walk-in clinic on 2 occasions and both times treated for bronchitis, first with amoxicillin and later with moxifloxacin without any clinical improvement. The patient is a nonsmoker. He works at a family-owned automobile restoration store. Hobbies include fishing, boating, and golfing. He denies any risk factors for tuberculosis or infection with the human immunodeficiency virus.

On physical examination temperature is 36.7°C, respiratory rate is 20 breaths/min, heart rate is 84 beats/min, and blood pressure is 119/79 mm Hg. Digital clubbing is not present. Inspection of the thorax does not show any chest wall abnormalities. Resonance is normal with bimanual percussion. Auscultation of the lungs reveals bibasilar, early inspiratory fine crackles. Whispered and spoken syllables are not distinctly louder at the lung bases. A complete blood count with differential is normal. Posteroanterior and lateral view chest radiographs reveal bilateral peripheral areas of consolidation with air bronchograms present. Computed tomography scanning of the chest is performed. A representative image is shown in figure 52-A. Bronchoscopy with bronchoalveolar lavage in the superior section of the lingula is performed with the differential cell count showing 65% alveolar macrophages, 20% lymphocytes, 10% neutrophils, and 5% eosinophils. Microbiology studies for bacteria, fungi, and viruses are negative. The patient undergoes a video-assisted thoracoscopic surgery with biopsy of the left upper and lower lobes. A representative image is shown in figure 52-B.

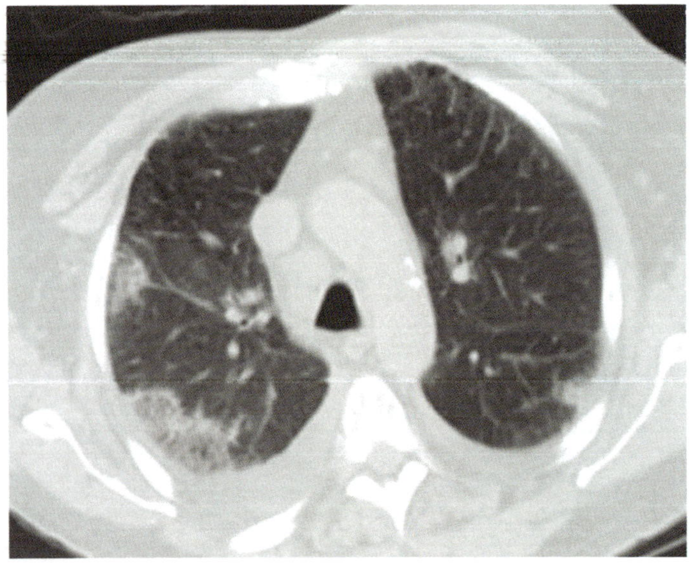

Figure 52-A

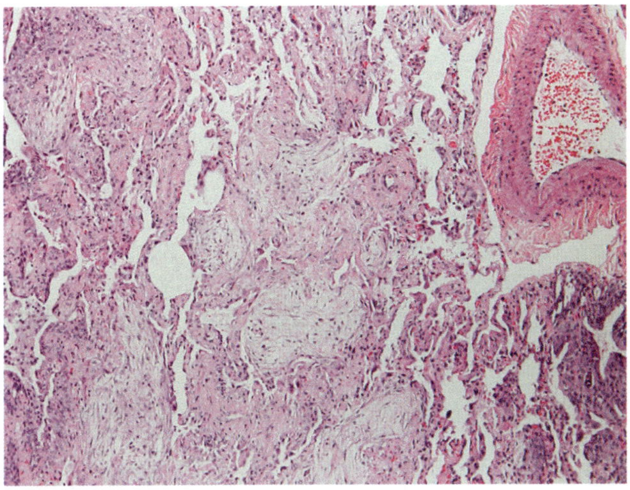

Figure 52-B

Which of the following statements about this condition is true?

A. Hemoptysis is a common presenting symptom.
B. The diagnosis can usually be made with a transbronchial biopsy.
C. The majority of patients respond poorly to prednisone.
D. Relapses are common but not associated with increased mortality or functional morbidity.

53. A 42-year-old female presents in the month of January with new onset fever and chills. She also complains of headache, muscle soreness involving the neck and shoulders, a nonproductive cough, and mild diarrhea. On physical examination temperature is 39.2°C, heart rate is 80 beats/min, respiratory rate is 22 breaths/min, and blood pressure is 134/82 mm Hg. The patient is alert and oriented. There is no nuchal rigidity. Pupils are equal in size and there is consensual reaction to light. Fundi are unremarkable. The heart rhythm is regular, and there are no murmurs. Auscultation of the lungs reveals bibasilar early inspiratory crackles. There is a diffuse, pale, macular rash present mostly involving the thorax and abdomen. The spleen tip is palpable. Posteroanterior and lateral view chest radiographs show bilateral densities in the lower lobes. Leukocyte count is 9,000/cu mm with 70% segmented neutrophils, 10% band forms, and 20% lymphocytes. BUN is 21 mg/dL, creatinine is 1.6 mg/dL, and sodium is 133 mEq/L. Liver function tests are normal. The patient is treated with doxycycline and makes a complete recovery.

Which one of the following statements about this condition is true?

A. The patient has contact with birds.
B. Penicillin would have been equally effective.
C. In the Northern Hemisphere, the peak incidence occurs during the winter months.
D. Nosocomial infections may occur if the offending organism colonizes the water supply.

54. A 24-year-old female has not felt well for the past 3 months. She initially experienced fatigue, low-grade fevers, muscle soreness, and a 12-pound weight loss. This was followed by shortness of breath, nonproductive cough, and pleurisy. A review of systems is positive for pain involving the knees, wrists, and proximal joints in her fingers. Ankles, shoulders, and hip joints are not involved.

On physical examination temperature is 37.8°C, blood pressure is 150/90 mm Hg, heart rate is 74 beats/min, and respiratory rate is 20 breaths/min. The rhythm and amplitude of respiration appear normal. No chest wall deformities are evident upon inspection of the thorax. There is dullness to percussion at the lung bases. Auscultation reveals diminished breath sounds at the bases. Whispered and spoken syllables are decreased. The remainder of the exam is notable for tenderness involving the proximal interphalangeal joints of the fingers on both hands. Hemoglobin is 11 g/dL, erythrocyte sedimentation rate is 53 mm/hr, C3 is 84 mg/dL, C4 is 9 mg/dL, ANA is >1:320, antibodies to double-stranded DNA are 40%, and antistreptolysin O titer is 150 Todd units. Chest radiographs show small bilateral pleural effusions with a normal cardiac silhouette. A diagnostic thoracentesis is performed.

Which one of the following statements about this condition is true?
A. A pleural fluid ANA > 1:40 is considered diagnostic.
B. The pleural fluid indices are likely to have exudative characteristics.
C. A reoccurring moderate to large unilateral pleural effusion frequently complicates the course.
D. Pleurodesis is typically required for long-term management.

55. A 52-year-old male with a history of very severe chronic obstructive pulmonary disease underwent a single lung transplant 13 months ago. Over the past 6 weeks, he has noticed worsening shortness of breath and dry cough. Current medications are prednisone, tacrolimus, and azathioprine. Computed tomography scanning of the chest shows multiple nodules in the lung allograft. The largest nodule measures approximately 1.5 cm in greatest diameter. A percutaneous core biopsy of this lesion is performed. The histopathology shows a polyclonal lymphoid proliferation. The B-cell lymphocytes have normal cytogenetics.

Which one of the following should be performed?
A. Administer cyclophosphamide, doxorubicin, vincristine, and prednisone followed by radiation to the involved field.
B. Substitute mycophenolate mofetil for azathioprine while continuing prednisone and tacrolimus.
C. Continue prednisone, tacrolimus, and azathioprine but all at reduced dosages.
D. Begin intravenous ganciclovir.

56. A 23-year-old male college student is admitted to the hospital with hemoptysis. He first noted the onset of a cough approximately 2 weeks ago. Over the last several days he has brought up increasing amounts of bright red blood. He is aware of some breathlessness with exertion. He denies fevers, chills, sweating, chest pain, blood in his urine, skin rash, or joint discomfort. He has no history of chronic illnesses or prior surgeries. His only habit is smoking 1 pack of cigarettes daily. He does not consume alcohol or use illicit drugs. Family history is positive for coronary artery disease in his father and asthma in 2 siblings.

On physical examination temperature is 37°C, heart rate is 110 beats/min, blood pressure is 135/82 mm Hg, and respiratory rate is 23 breaths/min. Room air oxygen saturation measured by pulse oximeter is 91%. He is alert and oriented. He appears mildly uncomfortable but is in no distress. Auscultation of the heart demonstrates a normal S1 and S2 without any summation gallop or murmur. Lung sounds are clear bilaterally. Liver edge and spleen tip are not felt. Extremities are warm without any clubbing, cyanosis, or peripheral edema. Chest radiographs show patchy air space disease bilaterally. Hemoglobin is 11 g/dL, with an MCV of 79 fL. Creatinine is 3.1 mg/dL, BUN is 38 mg/dL, and bicarbonate is 21 mEq/L. Microscopic urine analysis shows dysmorphic red blood cells and occasional red blood cell casts.

The morning following admission the patient undergoes an ultrasound-guided percutaneous biopsy of the right kidney. The histology specimen shows focal segmental necrotizing glomerulonephritis with crescent formation. There is linear deposition of immunoglobulin and complement along the basement membrane. His clinical condition is unchanged from the time of admission. He is producing approximately 30 mL/hr of urine.

Which of the following treatments should be started?

A. Plasmapheresis.
B. Plasmapheresis and prednisone.
C. Plasmapheresis, prednisone, and cyclophosphamide.
D. Hemodialysis, prednisone, and cyclophosphamide.

57. A 72-year-old female is experiencing hand weakness, right foot drop, dyspnea with exertion, orthopnea, and insomnia. She has no symptoms of dysphagia, dysarthria, or drooling. On physical examination there is evidence of muscle atrophy in the hands. Muscle fasciculations and hyperreflexia are also present. Tongue movements, extraocular muscles, and speech are normal. Affect is appropriate. A supine FVC is less than 50% of predicted.

Which statement about the use of noninvasive positive pressure ventilation (NIPPV) in patients with this condition is true?

A. Use of NIPPV for greater than 4 hours/day will have no effect on the rate of FVC decline.
B. Early institution of NIPPV may result in an improvement in the quality of life and a survival benefit.
C. NIPPV is contraindicated.
D. The benefit is greatest in individuals with severe bulbar dysfunction.

58. A 35-year-old female presents with worsening dyspnea on exertion and a cough productive of white sputum. Symptoms developed several months ago and have slowly progressed. She denies chest pain, wheezing, and hemoptysis. She is married and stays at home with her 2 young children. Past medical history is remarkable for oculocutaneous albinism, bruising, and menorrhagia. She is on no medications and does not smoke. She is unaware of her family history since she was adopted.

On physical examination the patient appears mildly uncomfortable but is in no distress. Respiratory rate is 24 breaths/min. Hair and skin are fair. Auscultation of the lungs reveals bilateral lower lobe early inspiratory fine crackles that do not clear with coughing. Digital clubbing is not present. Pulmonary function tes shows a total lung capacity of 64% of predicted and a diffusion capacity of 62% of predicted. The FEV_1/FVC ratio is 90%. Complete blood count and complete metabolic panel are normal. Posteroanterior and lateral view chest radiographs show diffuse bilateral interstitial infiltrates with a predilection for the basilar regions.

A surgical biopsy of the lung will show which one of the following histological abnormalities?

A. Interstitial smooth muscle proliferation with thin-walled cysts.
B. Diffuse uniform alveolar septal thickening with hyaline membranes. Granulomas and eosinophils are absent.
C. Type II epithelial cell hyperplasia with bland pulmonary hemorrhage. There is destruction of alveolar structures.
D. Areas of normal lung alternating with areas of dense collagen, scattered foci of fibrotic proliferation, and cystic fibrotic air spaces. Hyaline membranes are absent.

59. An act of bioterrorism occurs in a crowded subway station of a large metropolitan city. Over the next 3–10 days, several emergency rooms see patients with a syndrome that initially started with fever, chills, headache, and myalgias, followed by a cough and difficulty breathing. Chest radiographs show diffuse bilateral alveolar densities. Laboratory data shows lymphopenia, thrombocytopenia, and an elevated lactate dehydrogenase.

Which one of the following biological agents is the most likely cause of this illness?

A. Coronavirus.
B. Hantavirus.
C. Influenza A virus.
D. Adenovirus.

60. A 40-year-old female with a history of asthma is experiencing increasing respiratory symptoms. About 5 times in the last month she has awoken from sleep with wheezing, coughing, and breathlessness. She had similar symptoms on 2 occasions while at work in the past week. Every episode has improved with use of a short-acting beta agonist rescue inhaler. Past medical history includes endometriosis and gastroesophageal reflux controlled with diet modification and elevation of the head of the bed with 6-inch blocks. Current medications are oral ethinyl estradiol/drospirenone and pirbuterol meter dose inhaler.

On physical examination vital signs are stable. The patient is in no distress. There are no wheezes appreciated with auscultation of the lungs. Spirometry performed in the office reveals an FEV_1 of 85% of predicted. The FEV_1/FVC ratio is 82%.

Which one of the following should be performed next?

A. Schedule ciclesonide 80 mcg two inhalations twice daily.
B. Schedule pirbuterol two inhalations 10 minutes before bedtime and every 4-6 hours as needed.
C. Schedule ranitidine 300 mg before bedtime.
D. Schedule omeprazole 20 mg one hour before the evening meal.

61. A primary care clinic recently acquired a spirometer to use in the evaluation of patients with respiratory symptoms. Which statement about the diagnosis and management of chronic obstructive pulmonary disease is true?

A. Asymptomatic individuals with evidence of fixed airflow obstruction should be treated with an inhaled long-acting anticholinergic agent or an inhaled long-acting beta agonist.
B. Spirometry should be used as a screening test for airflow obstruction in asymptomatic patients at risk for chronic obstructive pulmonary disease.
C. Communication of spirometry results to patients leads to an increase in smoking cessation.
D. Periodic spirometry after initiation of therapy should not be used to monitor disease status in stable patients.

62. A 70-year-old female is admitted to the hospital with chest pain. She was in her usual state of health until about one week ago when she developed a flu-like illness. She felt feverish with diffuse body aches, runny nose, sore throat, hoarse voice, and productive cough. She spent the next several days convalescing at home. Her condition seemed to be gradually improving when she developed sudden chest pain this morning prompting her to seek medical attention. She describes the pain as located over the anterior chest and worse with deep inspiration and coughing. At times it radiates into both shoulders. Past medical history includes hypertension, diabetes mellitus, and mild obstructive sleep apnea treated with a mandibular advancement device. Current medications are amlodipine, glipizide, aspirin, calcium, and vitamin D.

On physical examination the patient is lying in bed and appears uncomfortable. Temperature is 38.3°C, heart rate is 105 beats/min, blood pressure measured in the right arm is 140/85 mm Hg with no pulsus paradoxus, and respiratory rate is 20 breaths/min. Jugular venous pulsations appear normal. Inspection, percussion, and palpation of the precordium are unremarkable. With the patient leaning forward, auscultation with the stethoscope diaphragm reveals a scratchy noise best heard between the apex of the heart and sternum at end expiration. No cardiac murmurs or gallops are present. Vesicular breath sounds are appreciated at the peripheries of both lungs. Chest radiographs do not show any parenchymal opacities or pleural effusions. Serum creatinine is 1.9 mg/dL, creatinine kinase is 24 U/L, total MB isoenzymes are 3 U/L, and a D-dimer is 500 ng/mL.

Which one of the following tests will lead to a correct diagnosis?

A. Pulmonary angiogram.
B. Ventilation profusion scanning.
C. Electrocardiogram.
D. Computerized tomography scanning of the chest following administration of intravenous contrast.

63. A 72-year-old male presents with fatigue, anorexia, and weakness. He describes difficulty climbing up a flight of steps. A review of systems is positive for recent onset dry mouth, constipation, and muscle cramping. He takes allopurinol for gout and hydrochlorothiazide for hypertension. He has a 42-pack-year history of smoking cigarettes.

On physical examination temperature is 37.4°C, heart rate is 91 beats/min, blood pressure is 132/92 mm Hg, and respiratory rate is 20 breaths/min. There is slight drooping of the left upper eyelid. Extraocular muscles appear intact. Pupils are equal in size but reaction to light is sluggish. Cardiopulmonary examination is unremarkable. There is symmetric weakness involving the proximal muscles of the lower extremities. Patellar tendon reflexes are decreased. There is no evidence of paradoxical abdominal motion with breathing while the patient is in the supine position.

Chest radiographs show a peripheral right upper lobe pulmonary nodule. Computed tomography scanning of the chest is performed. A representative image is shown in figure 63-A. A biopsy is performed. A representative image is shown in figure 63-B.

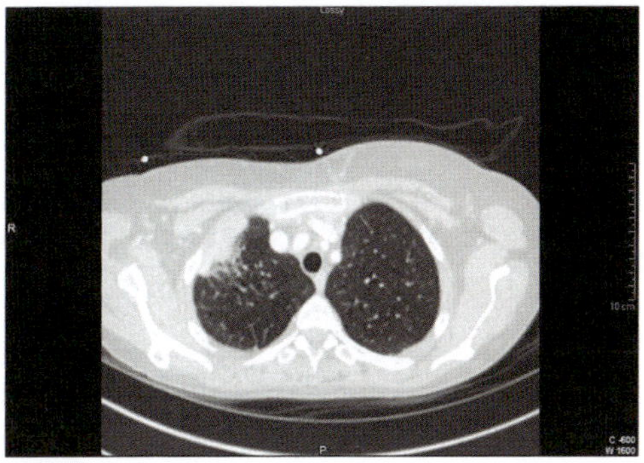

Figure 63-A

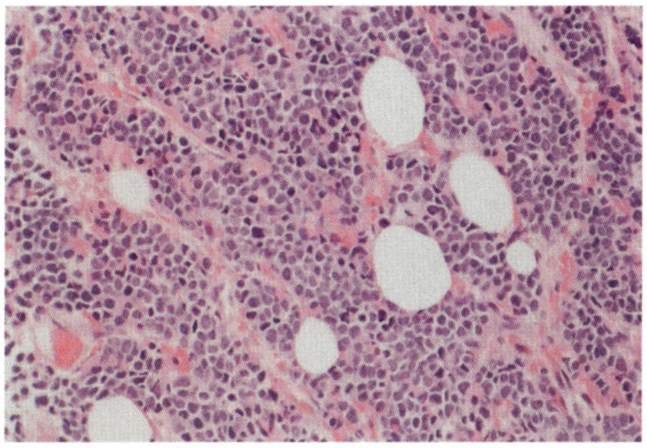

Figure 63-B

Which one of the following about the patient's condition is false?

A. Repetitive nerve stimulation of an involved muscle will show an increase in the compound muscle action potential.
B. Repetitive nerve stimulation of an involved muscle will show a decrease in the compound muscle action potential.
C. The serum antibody titer against P/Q-type voltage-gated calcium channel will be high.
D. Isometric contractions of an involved muscle will lead to transient improvement in muscle strength.

64. A 31-year-old male presents to the emergency room with a 3-day history of fever, shortness of breath, and cough. He was in his usual state of health until prior to this. Past medical history includes depression for which he takes mirtazapine. He smokes approximately 1 pack of cigarettes per day. He is a graduate student in biochemistry at the local university. He denies owning any pets, recent travel history, or risk factors for infection with the human immunodeficiency virus.

On physical examination temperate is 38°C, heart rate is 115 beats/min, blood pressure is 180/90 mm Hg, and respiratory rate is 28 breaths/min. Oxygen saturation measured by pulse oximetry while breathing ambient air is 78% and improves to 90% with administration of 6 L/min of supplemental oxygen. Auscultation of the lungs reveals early inspiratory crackles diffusely. The remainder of the exam is unremarkable. Leukocyte count is 12,000/cu mm, with 70% segmented neutrophils, 7% band forms, 20% lymphocytes, and 3% eosinophils. A portable anteroposterior view chest radiograph shows diffuse bilateral opacities.

Because of impending respiratory failure, the patient undergoes endotracheal intubation with initiation of mechanical ventilation. Antimicrobial therapy with intravenous vancomycin, ceftriaxone, and doxycycline is administered. Thirty-six hours later, the patient's condition is not improving. Bronchoscopy with bronchoalveolar lavage is performed in the medial segment of the right middle lobe. A representative image is shown in figure 64-A. Giemsa, acid-fast, and potassium hydroxide-treated smears are negative. No intranuclear or cytoplasmic inclusion bodies are identified. The patient is started on intravenous methylprednisolone 125 mg every 6 hours. He is successfully liberated from the ventilator 48 hours later.

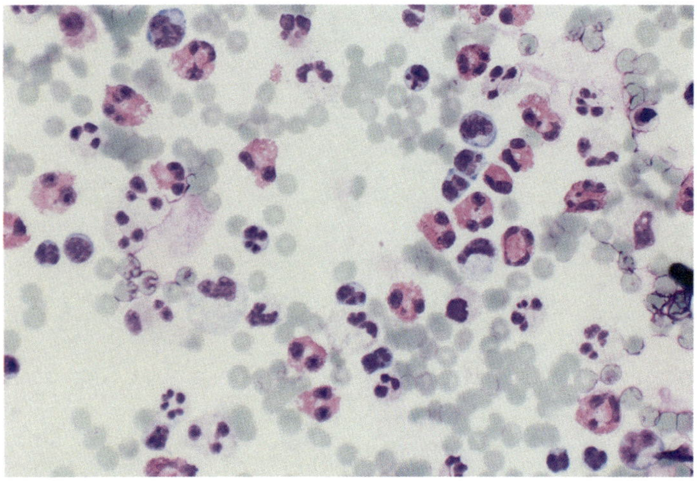

Figure 64-A

Which one of the following statements about this condition is true?

A. Cigarette smoking has been established as a causative agent.

B. The majority of patients have a history of asthma.

C. Relapse is common.

D. Stool analysis will reveal thick-shelled eggs.

65. A 22-year-old male who resides in Southern California is referred for evaluation. He was well until approximately 3 months ago. At that time, he developed an illness characterized by fever, cough, pleurisy, fatigue, and arthralgias. He sought medical attention at a local emergency room where chest radiography was performed. This demonstrated a patchy opacity in the left upper lobe with fullness in the left hilum. Leukocyte count was 12,000/cu mm with 65% segmented neutrophils, 27% lymphocytes, and 8% eosinophils. He was treated with doxycycline for presumed community-acquired pneumonia. A month later, he saw his primary care physician for follow up. The patient felt well, but repeat chest radiographs now showed a 2-cm thin-walled cavity in the left upper lobe. Physical examination is normal. Complete blood count and complete metabolic panel are normal. He denies risk factors for infection with the human immunodeficiency virus. He is a nonsmoker. Tuberculin skin test is nonreactive.

Which one of the following should be recommended?
A. Fluconazole 400 mg orally once a day for 3 months.
B. Itraconazole 400 mg orally once a day for 3 months.
C. Isoniazid, rifampin, ethambutol, and pyrazinamide for 8 weeks followed by isoniazid and rifampin for 16 weeks.
D. Observation.

66. A 36-year-old female with a history of asthma and allergic rhinitis is having problems with symptom control. She is currently taking fluticasone 500 mcg/salmeterol 50 mcg one inhalation twice daily, zafirlukast 20 mg orally twice daily, cetirizine 10 mg orally once a day, fluticasone nasal spray 2 sprays per nostril once daily and metaproterenol 2 inhalations every 6 hours as needed. She is interested in purchasing a high-efficiency particulate air (HEPA) filter.

Which one of the following statements about HEPA filters is false?
A. Reduces airborne dog and cat allergens.
B. Reduces airborne mold spores.
C. Reduces airborne dust mite and cockroach particles.
D. Reduces particulate tobacco smoke.

67. An 18-year-old female presents with cystic fibrosis. She has a chronic cough with daily sputum production. She denies hemoptysis. During a recent hospitalization for a pulmonary exacerbation, a sputum culture grew mucoid *Pseudomonas aeruginosa.*

On physical examination the patient is thin and in no distress. Temperature is 36.9°C, heart rate is 92 beats/min, blood pressure is 118/60 mm Hg, and respiratory rate is 20 breaths/min. Oxygen saturation measured by pulse oximetry performed on room air is 94%. Digital clubbing is present. Inspection of the thorax is notable for a slight left thoracic curvature. Percussion demonstrates hyperresonance. With auscultation, whispered pectoriloquy and bronchophony are indistinctly heard. Bilateral end expiratory wheezes are appreciated. Posteroanterior and lateral view chest radiographs show a normal-size cardiac silhouette, hyperinflation, and increased linear markings in the upper lobes bilaterally. Leukocyte count is 9,000/cu mm with 70% segmented neutrophils, 3% band forms, 2% eosinophils, and 25% lymphocytes. IgE is 300 IU/mL. Immediate skin prick testing to *Aspergillus fumigatus* is negative. A postbronchodilator FEV_1 is 48% of predicted.

Which one of the following should not be used in the management of this patient?
A. A high-frequency chest wall oscillation system.
B. Nebulized dornase alpha once daily.
C. Beta-2 adrenergic receptor agonist nebulized every 4-6 hours.
D. An oral glucocorticoid once daily.

68. An 18-year-old female with sickle cell anemia is admitted to the hospital with chest pain, cough, fever, and shortness of breath. On physical examination the patient appears mildly uncomfortable. Temperature is 39.1°C, heart rate is 110 beats/min, blood pressure is 140/85 mm Hg, and respiratory rate is 26 breaths/min. Oxygen saturation measured by pulse oximetry is 91% while breathing room air. Precordial palpation is positive for a thrust between the apex and the sternum at the 4th interspace. Auscultation of the heart reveals a prominent P_2 sound. Lung sounds are positive for bibasilar fine crackles at end inspiration. Whispered and spoken syllables are not distinct. Posteroanterior and lateral view chest radiographs show bibasilar infiltrates. Laboratory data is remarkable for a hemoglobin of 7.8 g/dL, leukocyte count of 21,000/cu mm with 80% segmented neutrophils, and a platelet count of 190,000/cu mm.

All of the following interventions would be appropriate except which one?
A. Have the patient perform frequent bedside incentive spirometry.
B. Begin antibiotic therapy with intravenous vancomycin.
C. Transfuse with red blood cells to achieve a hemoglobin level of 10 g/dL.
D. Administer supplemental oxygen to keep pulse oximeter higher than 92%.

69. An 82-year-old retired female optometrist presents with worsening shortness of breath and a nonproductive cough. Symptoms developed approximately 4 months ago and have gradually progressed. A review of systems is otherwise negative. Past medical history includes hypertension, gout, a positive tuberculin skin test, and paroxysmal atrial fibrillation. Current medications are amiodarone 200 mg orally once daily, warfarin 5 mg orally once daily, allopurinol 100 mg orally once daily, and losartan 25 mg once daily.

Physical examination is unremarkable. Complete blood count with differential, blood urea nitrogen, and creatinine are within normal ranges. Chest radiographs show a 3 cm opacity in the left upper lobe. The lesion is new when compared to a prior study done 6 months ago when the atrial arrhythmia was diagnosed. Chest computed tomography scan with contract shows a 3 cm irregular mass in the anterior segment of the left upper lobe. There is no associated mediastinal adenopathy. Bronchoscopy with bronchoalveolar lavage and transbronchial biopsies is nondiagnostic. The patient undergoes a video-assisted thoracoscopic lung biopsy. A representative image is shown in figure 69-A. Special stains for fungi and acid-fast bacilli are negative.

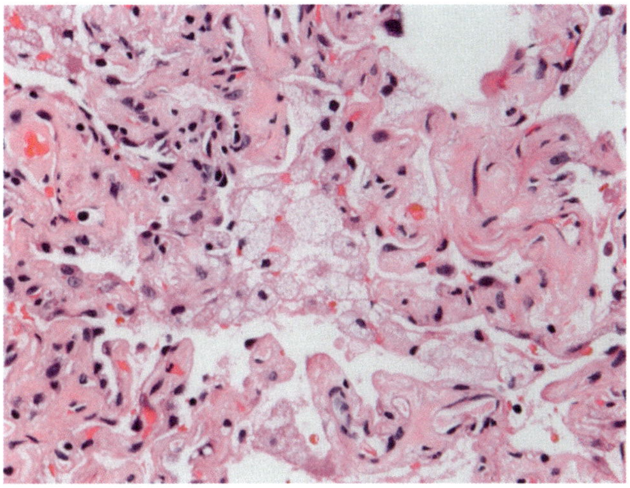

Figure 69-A

Which one of the following should be performed next?

A. Begin isoniazid, rifampin, ethambutol, and pyrazinamide.
B. Discontinue amiodarone.
C. Left upper lobectomy.
D. Begin prednisone 1 mg/kg per day.

70. A 43-year-old male seeks medical attention for progressive shortness of breath and cough. Symptoms have been present for the past several months. Physical examination is notable only for high-pitched midinspiratory squeaks heard during auscultation of the lungs. Pulmonary function test shows severe fixed airway obstruction with air trapping and a diffusion capacity that is normal. Chest radiographs suggests hyperinflation. A high-resolution computed tomography scan of the chest is performed at end expiration. There are multiple areas of decreased attenuation and vascularity with evidence of air trapping. Some of the bronchioles have thickened walls and appear dilated. A thoracoscopic lung biopsy is performed. The findings show complete obliteration of the airway lumen with a relatively unremarkable appearance of the distal alveoli.

A detailed occupational history would reveal that this patient was most likely exposed to which one of the following?

A. Isocyanates.
B. Thermophilic actinomycetes.
C. Nitrogen dioxide.
D. Bird protein antigen.

71. A 66-year-old male presents with a 3-day history of fever, chills, sweats, and a cough productive of yellowish phlegm. On physical examination temperature is 39.1°C, heart rate is 102 beats/min, respiratory rate is 24 breaths/min, and blood pressure is 120/65 mm Hg. He is alert and oriented. Inspection of the thorax is unremarkable. The rhythm and amplitude of his respirations are normal. Over the right mid-chest, vibratory palpation is increased. Bimanual palpation in this area reveals medium intensity dullness. Auscultation of the lungs is positive for fine crackles at end inspiration in the right mid-lung. Whispered and spoken syllables are clear over this region. Leukocyte count is 15,000/cu mm with 75% segmented neutrophils, 7% band forms, and 23% lymphocytes. Creatinine is 1.0 mg/dL and BUN is 21 mg/dL. Chest radiographs are obtained and shown in figures 71-A and 71-B.

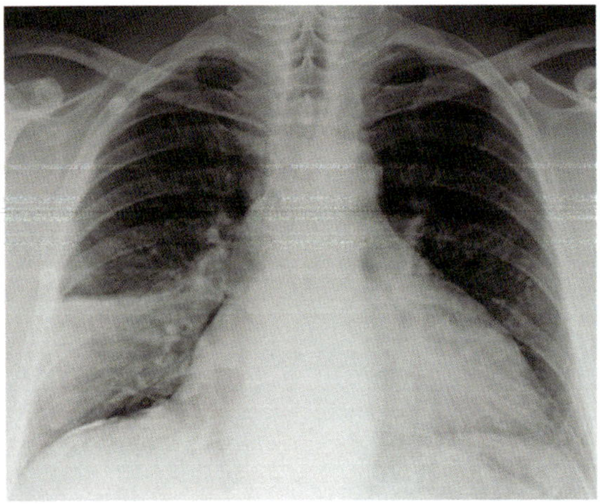

Figure 71-A

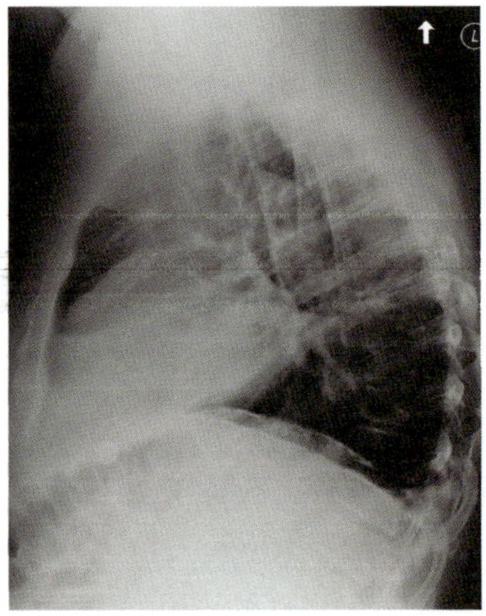

Figure 71-B

Which one of the following is the most appropriate disposition?

A. Discharge to home on oral doxycycline.
B. Discharge to home on oral levofloxacin.
C. Admission to the hospital general medical ward and start oral levofloxacin.
D. Admission to the intensive care unit and start intravenous cefepime and levofloxacin.

72. A 76-year-old male complains of recent onset right-sided chest discomfort. Past medical history includes hypertension, nonocclusive coronary artery disease, and allergic rhinitis. He denies shortness of breath, cough, fever, and weight loss. Electrocardiogram shows normal sinus rhythm. Chest radiographs show a moderate-size left pleural effusion. Computed tomography scanning of the chest is performed. A representative image is shown in figure 72-A. He is a lifelong nonsmoker. After briefly serving in the military, he was a family law attorney until his retirement a decade ago.

A diagnostic thoracentesis is performed. Approximately 1 liter of bloody fluid is removed. The pleural fluid cell count is 2,500 nucleated cells/ microL with 35% polymorphonuclear cells, 45% lymphocytes, and 20% eosinophils. Fluid LDH is 175 U/L and protein 4 g/dL. Simultaneous serum LDH is 265 U/L and total protein 7.8 g/dL. Cytologic analysis does not show any malignant cells. The smear for acid-fast bacilli is negative and the culture shows no growth to date. Follow-up chest radiographs performed 3 weeks later show a persistent small left effusion.

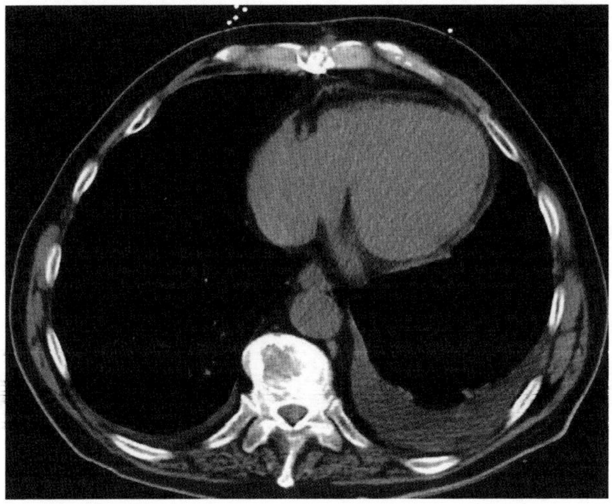

Figure 72-A

Which one of the following should be performed next?
A. Take additional occupational history.
B. Administer isoniazid, rifampin, ethambutol, and pyrazinamide.
C. Video-assisted thoracoscopic surgery with pleural biopsy.
D. Video-assisted thoracoscopic surgery with pleural biopsy and intraoperative peurodesis.

73. An 80-year-old male is admitted to the hospital with fever and chest pain that radiates to the neck and shoulders. One month ago, he underwent 4-vessel coronary artery bypass grafting for symptomatic coronary artery disease. He had an uncomplicated hospital course and was discharged to home on the 5th postoperative day. He is attending cardiac rehabilitation 2 days per week. His postoperative course has been unremarkable until now. He is a nonsmoker. Current medications include aspirin, carvedilol, simvastatin, lisinopril, and furosemide.

On physical examination temperature is 38.6°C, heart rate is 92 beats/min, and respiratory rate is 20 breaths/min. Blood pressure in the right arm is 135/80 mm Hg, and the change in arterial systolic pressure with inspiration is only 7 mm Hg. Examination of the thorax reveals a well-healed sternotomy scar. Auscultation of the anterior chest using the diaphragm of the stethoscope reveals a scratchy noise best heard over the left sternal border at end expiration. It intensifies when the patient leans forward. Breath sounds are clear except for an area that is diminished at the left base. There is associated dullness with percussion over this area, but no egophony. With the patient seated at a 45° angle, examination of the external jugular veins show normal x and y descents. There is no venous distention appreciated with inspiration. Chest radiographs show a normal-size cardiac silhouette and a small left pleural effusion with an adjacent parenchymal density. Leukocyte count is 14,000/cu mm with a normal differential. Blood, urine, and sputum cultures for bacteria are negative.

Which one of the following statements about this condition is true?

A. Chest tube thoracostomy should be performed.
B. Catheter pericardiocentesis should be performed.
C. Administration of colchicine postoperatively may have prevented this illness.
D. Administration of indomethacin postoperatively may have prevented this illness.

74. A 38-year-old male is postoperative day 6 after autologous hematopoietic stem cell transplantation for chronic myelogenous leukemia when he develops progressive shortness of breath, cough, and hypoxemia. There is no hemoptysis, fevers, chills, or sweats.

On physical examination temperature is 36.9° C, respiratory rate is 28 breaths/min, heart rate is 113 beats/min, and blood pressure is 146/89 mm Hg. Oxygen saturation measured by pulse oximetry is 92% while the patient receives 6 L/min of supplemental oxygen via nasal cannula. Cutaneous examination is positive for scattered ecchymosis and generalized alopecia. The oropharynx is notable for mucositis. Lung sounds are clear to auscultation. Heart tones are regular and no gallops are present. Chest radiographs show multiple patchy alveolar densities. Bronchoscopy is performed with bronchoalveolar lavage in the inferior segment of the lingula. Sequential aliquots are progressively bloodier.

Which one of the following statements about this condition is false?
A. The incidence appears to be similar among autologous and allogenic recipients.
B. Thrombocytopenia is not a risk factor for this condition.
C. Most cases present within the first month after transplantation.
D. Death is usually due to refractory pulmonary hemorrhage.

75. The most common pathogen responsible for pulmonary exacerbations in adults with cystic fibrosis is:
A. *Pseudomonas aeruginosa.*
B. *Burkholderia cepacia.*
C. *Staphylococcus aureus.*
D. *Haemophilus influenzae.*

76. How long should montelukast be held prior to performing a bronchoprovocation test with methacholine?
A. 24 hours.
B. 48 hours.
C. 72 hours.
D. 1 week.

77. A 31-year-old female has been experiencing progressive dyspnea with exertion over the last 6 months (New York Heart Association Functional Class I). She was originally treated for presumed asthma with a prolonged course of an inhaled glucocorticoid and a short-acting beta agonist without any improvement. She denies chest pain, syncope, cough, or wheezing. She has never taken any anorexigen drugs. ANA titer is 1:40. Enzyme immunoassay screening for antibodies against the human immunodeficiency virus is negative.

On physical examination the patient is afebrile, heart rate is 74 beats/min, blood pressure is 119/73 mm Hg, and respiratory rate is 20 breaths/min. Oxygen saturation measured by pulse oximetry is 93% on room air. With the diaphragm of the stethoscope placed over the left 2nd intercostal space, the 2nd heart sound is accentuated and split. A prominent a wave is appreciated upon inspection of the neck veins. There is trace pedal edema. Electrocardiogram shows right axis deviation and an increase in the P-wave amplitude in lead II. Chest radiographs show enlarged pulmonary arteries without any parenchymal or pleural changes. Transthoracic echocardiography with Doppler ultrasound estimates the pulmonary arterial systolic pressure at greater than 50 mm Hg. Right heart catheterization is performed. Pulmonary capillary wedge pressure is 10 mm Hg. Mean pulmonary arterial pressure is 44 mg Hg. A vasoreactivity test is performed using intravenous adenosine. The mean pulmonary arterial pressure decreases to 32 mm Hg, and there is no change in the cardiac output.

Which one of the following should be initiated?
A. Verapamil.
B. Amlodipine and warfarin.
C. Intravenous epoprostenol.
D. Inhaled iloprost.

78. A 77-year-old male was in his usual state of health until approximately 6 months ago when he developed left shoulder pain. He sought medical attention with his primary health care provider and was diagnosed with subacromial bursitis. The pain did not resolve with nonsteroidal anti-inflammatory medications or an injection of methylprednisolone/lidocaine into the bursa. When the pain started to radiate into the neck and left arm, radiographs of the shoulder were performed. Incidentally identified was a left apical lung mass.

On physical examination vital signs are stable. There is anisocoria with the left more miotic. The palpebral fissure is narrower on the left. Heart tones are normal, and lung sounds are clear bilaterally. There is mild atrophy noted along the 4th and 5th digits of the left hand. Motor testing reveals mild weakness of the intrinsic muscles of the left hand. Inspection and palpation of the left shoulder are normal. There is full range of active and passive motion.

Which one of the following is true?
A. Biopsy of the mass will most likely reveal a small-cell lung cancer.
B. The primary tumor is a T3 lesion.
C. Magnetic resonance imaging is superior to computed tomography for detecting tumor involvement of the brachial plexus.
D. Combined radiotherapy and extended surgical resection results in a 5-year survival rate of close to 50%.

79. A 62-year-old male who works for the Department of Corrections presents with progressive shortness of breath and a nonproductive cough. Physical examination is notable for digital clubbing and early bibasilar inspiratory crackles. Chest radiographs show curvilinear densities at the lung bases. A high-resolution computed tomography scan of the chest is performed. Representative images are shown in figures 79-A and 79-B. The patient undergoes video-assisted thoracoscopic biopsy. A representative image is shown in figure 79-C.

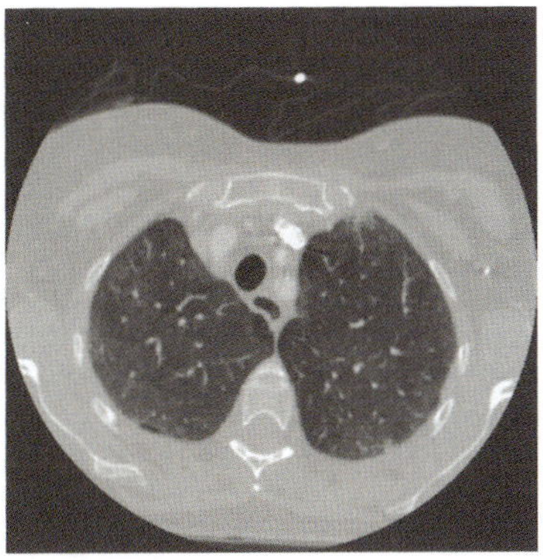

Figure 79-A

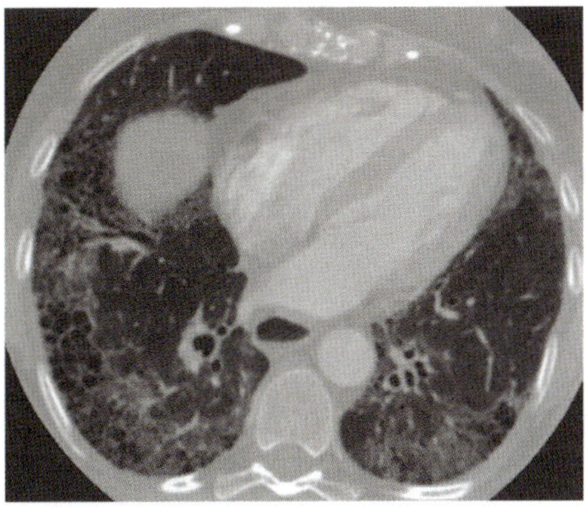

Figure 79-B

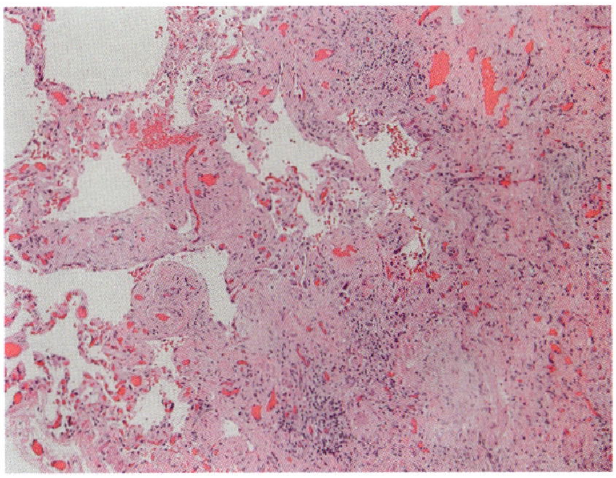

Figure 79-C

Which one of the following baseline studies in this condition is not associated with an increased risk of subsequent mortality?

A. Diffusion capacity for carbon monoxide less than 40% of predicated.
B. Extent of honeycombing on high-resolution computed tomography scan.
C. Mean pulmonary artery pressure of greater than 25 mm Hg at rest.
D. Forced vital capacity less than 65% of predicted.

80. A 52-year-old male complains of chronic shortness of breath with exertion that is progressively getting worse. A review of systems is positive for fatigue, malaise, and bilateral ankle swelling. He denies cough, wheezing, or chest pain. On physical examination the patient is in no distress. Percussion of the precordium shows a maximum intensity between the left 2nd and 3rd ribs. A precordial thrust to the right of this can be palpated. P_2 is accentuated. A basal diastolic murmur is appreciated. A holosystolic murmur that increases with deep inspiration is also present. With the patient reclining at 45°, jugular venous pulsations are appreciated 6 cm above the sternal angle. Examination of the abdomen reveals a palpable liver edge 4 cm below the right rib margin. There is dullness to percussion over the left upper quadrant near the anterior axillary line. The flanks are not bulging, and there is no evidence of shifting dullness. There is mild pitting edema involving both ankles.

The patient claims to otherwise be healthy except for an isolated illness that occurred approximately 25 years ago in his homeland of Egypt. As a young man, he frequently went swimming and even bathed in fresh water. After one episode of swimming, he developed a particularly bothersome pruritic rash. Five weeks later, he had an illness characterized by fever, lethargy, sweats, diarrhea, severe cough, and shortness of breath. He never sought medical attention for this.

Which one of the following organisms is most likely responsible for the patient's presentation?
A. *Schistosoma mansoni.*
B. *Echinococcus multilocularis.*
C. *Strongyloides stercoralis.*
D. *Plasmodium falciparum.*

81. A 62-year-old female seeks medical attention for a cough that has been present for approximately 1 year. She denies nasal congestion, postnasal drip, pain with swallowing, difficulty swallowing, weight loss, change in voice, or sore throat. The cough is nonproductive. There is no associated wheezing or shortness of breath. Her primary care physician treated her for presumed asthma with a trial of a short-acting inhaled beta agonist without any symptom improvement. She was then referred to an allergist for evaluation. Skin testing and computed tomography scanning of the sinuses were nondiagnostic. She is currently not taking any medications. She is a lifelong nonsmoker. She is presently unemployed, having worked retail jobs in the past. Her only hobby is gardening.

On physical examination respiratory rate is 16 breaths/min. Nasal mucosa is moist, and there is no evidence of cobblestoning in the oropharynx. No stridor is appreciated with auscultation over the trachea. Lung sounds are clear bilaterally. Posteroanterior and lateral view chest radiographs demonstrate a normal-size cardiac silhouette and no evidence of pleural effusions or parenchymal infiltrates. Bronchoprovocation testing with methacholine fails to show a drop in the FEV_1 after a total methacholine concentration of 16 mg/ml.

Which one of the following should be performed next?
A. Flexible bronchoscopy.
B. Induce sputum for differential cell count.

C. High-resolution computed tomography scanning of the chest.
D. Esophagoscopy.

82. Which one of the following is the most common genetic disease affecting the Caucasian population in the United States?
A. Alpha-1-antitrypsin deficiency.
B. Hereditary hemorrhagic telangiectasia.
C. Cystic fibrosis.
D. Tuberous sclerosis.

83. A 19-year-old male is seeking genetic counseling. His father died suddenly from an aortic dissection at age 42 years.

On physical examination the patient has evidence of a high-arched palate, down-slanting palpebral fissures, retrognathia, myopia, arachnodactyly, and mitral valve prolapse.

Which one of the following is the most common pulmonary complication accompanying this disorder?
A. Recurrent bronchopneumonia.
B. Pneumothorax.
C. Congenital absence of the right middle lobe.
D. Pulmonary artery aneurysm.

84. A 77-year-old male with a history of severe chronic obstructive pulmonary disease, hypertension, mild left ventricular dysfunction, and depression is admitted to the hospital with worsening shortness of breath, wheezing, and a cough productive of purulent sputum. Current medications include tiotropium one inhalation daily, albuterol metered dose inhaler two inhalations every 6 hours as needed, extended-release theophylline 400 mg orally once daily, digoxin 0.125 mg orally once daily, lisinopril 10 mg orally once daily, and citalopram 40 mg orally once daily.

Physical examination reveals an elderly male in mild distress. Temperature is 36.8°C, heart rate is 87 beats/min, respiratory rate is 28 breaths/min, and blood pressure is 135/68 mm Hg. Inspection of the thorax reveals a barrel-shaped chest. Expiration appears prolonged. Percussion of the chest does not demonstrate any areas of dullness or tympany. Auscultation of the lungs reveals bilateral expiratory wheezes diffusely. There is pitting edema involving both ankles. Posteroanterior and lateral view chest radiographs show hyperinflation without any infiltrates. Serum digoxin level is

1.0 ng/mL, theophylline level is 14 mcg/mL, sodium is 137 mEq/L, potassium is 3.7 mEq/L, chloride is 100 mEq/L, bicarbonate is 28 mEq/L, and a nonfasting glucose is 98 mg/dL. Treatment is initiated with intravenous methylprednisolone 40 mg every 8 hours, nebulized albuterol with ipratropium every 6 hours, and clarithromycin 500 mg orally twice daily.

On the 3rd hospital day the patient begins to experience insomnia, tachycardia, upper extremity tremor, abdominal discomfort, nausea, and agitation. On the 4th hospital day, the patient has a tonic-clonic seizure.

Which one of the following medications is responsible for the patient's deterioration?

A. Digoxin.
B. Ipratropium.
C. Theophylline.
D. Citalopram.

85. A 42-year-old single male presents with several months of progressive shortness of breath, cough, and fatigue. He denies fever, chest pain, and hemoptysis. Past medical history is unremarkable, and he denies use of illicit drugs, unprotected sexual activity, or exposure to individuals with tuberculosis. He is a host at a local restaurant, has no unusual hobbies, and owns no pets. He has a 20-pack-year history of smoking cigarettes.

On physical examination temperature is 38°C, respiratory rate 22 breaths/min, heart rate is 92 beats/min, and blood pressure is 123/74 mm Hg. Oxygen saturation measured by pulse oximetery on ambient air is 91%. There are no chest wall deformities upon inspection of the thorax. Auscultation of the lungs reveals bibasilar early inspiratory fine crackles. There is no evidence of digital clubbing, peripheral edema, joint deformity, or cutaneous rash. Leukocyte count is 12,500/cu mm with 60% segmented neutrophils, 35% lymphocytes, 5% eosinophils. Hemoglobin is 14 g/dL, platelet count is 350,000/cu mm, and LDH is 420 U/L. Liver function tests, renal indices, and urinalysis are unremarkable.

Posteroanterior and lateral view chest radiographs show bilateral diffuse symmetric alveolar opacities. Computed tomography scanning of the chest is performed. A representative image is shown in figure 85-A. Bronchoscopy with bronchoalveolar lavage and transbronchial biopsies is performed in the right middle lobe. The lavage fluid shows large amounts of acellular eosinophilic proteinaceous material with foamy macrophages. A representative image of a biopsy is shown in figure 85-B.

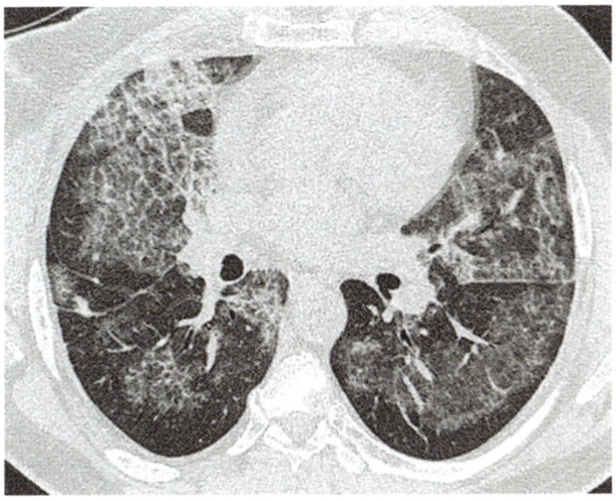

Figure 85-A

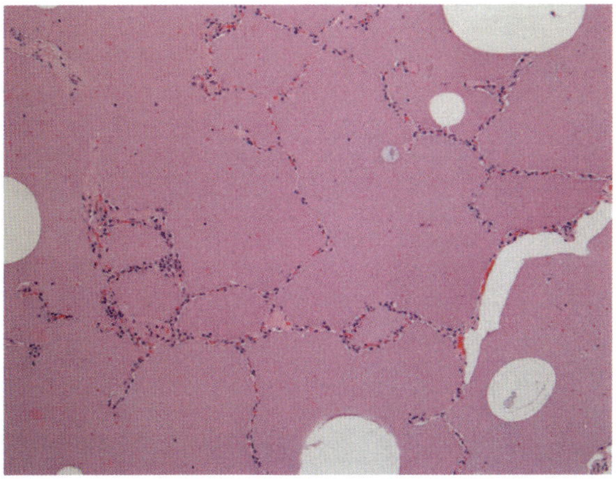

Figure 85-B

Which one of the following statements about this condition is true?

A. It usually occurs secondary to an underlying solid organ malignancy.
B. Trimethoprim-sulfasalazine should be started for prophylaxis against opportunistic infections.
C. All patients should undergo whole lung lavage.
D. In the acquired form, granulocyte macrophage-colony stimulating factor autoantibodies are present.

86. A 29-year-old male is being evaluated for fever, shortness of breath, and cough. Symptoms have been present for over 1 week. Past medical history is unremarkable except for an appendectomy at age 16. He is a second-generation dairy farmer in rural Iowa. Cattle and sheep are present on the property. He denies smoking cigarettes or consuming alcohol. He has been in a monogamous relationship with his male partner for the past 5 years.

On physical examination temperature is 40.1°C, heart rate is 62 beats/min, and respiratory rate is 20 breaths/min. The patient is alert, oriented, and in no distress. Mild conjunctivitis is present. Inspection and palpation of the thorax are unremarkable. Auscultation of the heart shows a normal S1 and S2 without any murmurs or gallops. Lung sounds are clear. Inspection of the abdomen reveals a right lower quadrant scar consistent with his prior appendectomy. The liver edge is palpable and feels smooth without any nodularity. There is no tenderness precipitated with fist percussion. The spleen tip can be felt below the left costal margin when the patient is instructed to take a deep breath. No cutaneous rash is present. Leukocyte count is 8,000/cu mm with a normal differential, hemoglobin is 15 g/dL, platelet count is 103,000/cu mm, ALT is 82 U/L, and AST is 90 U/L. Chest radiographs show a nodular infiltrate in the right middle lobe.

Which one of the following should be administered?
A. Streptomycin.
B. Doxycycline.
C. Azithromycin and rifampin.
D. Ceftriaxone and clarithromycin.

87. Which one of the following is the most common cause of community-acquired pneumonia in adults who do not require hospitalization?
A. *Streptococcus pneumoniae.*
B. *Haemophilus influenzae.*
C. *Mycoplasma pneumoniae.*
D. *Chlamydophila pneumoniae.*

88. Which one of the following is the most common cause of a nontraumatic chylothorax?
A. Lymphangioleiomyomatosis.
B. Small cell carcinoma.
C. Non-Hodgkin lymphoma.
D. Thoracic radiation.

89. Which one of the following patients would be at the lowest risk for postoperative pulmonary complications following an elective open repair of an abdominal aortic aneurysm?
A. A 53-year-old male with a body mass index of 40 kg/m^2.
B. A 53-year-old male with untreated obstructive sleep apnea (respiratory disturbance index 16/hr).
C. A 53-year-old male who smokes one pack of cigarettes a day. Postbronchodilator spirometry does not show fixed obstruction.
D. A 53-year-old male who smokes one pack of cigarettes a day. Postbronchodilator spirometry shows fixed moderate obstruction.

90. A 62-year-old male presents with acute hemoptysis. For the past 48 hours he has coughed up several teaspoons of bright red blood. He denies fever, chest pain, and shortness of breath. Past medical history includes epididymitis, apthous ulcers, arthritis, and intermittent pain in the right eye. Other than a once-a-day multivitamin he is on no medications. He denies smoking and has no risk factors for tuberculosis. Family history is unknown as both of his parents passed away shortly after immigrating to the United States from Turkey. He is the minister of a local parish.

On physical examination vital signs are stable. Examination of the oral cavity reveals multiple subcentimeter ulcers on the buccal mucosae. He has an extensive acneform rash on the face, chest, and back. Cardiac examination reveals a normal S1 and S2 without any gallop or murmur. Lung sounds are clear bilaterally. Passive movement of the left knee elicits mild pain. There is no evidence of joint deformity, erythema, or synovitis present. Leukocyte count is 13,000/cu mm with a normal differential, hemoglobin is 13.2 g/dL, platelet count is 390,000/cu mm, activated partial thromboplastin time is 32 seconds, and prothrombin time is 11 seconds. Chest radiographs show clear lung fields with a normal-size cardiac silhouette. No pleural effusions are present. As the patient is being prepared for diagnostic flexible bronchoscopy, he has an episode of massive hemoptysis and exsanguinates.

Which one of the following is most likely the cause of the patient's death?
A. Diffuse alveolar hemorrhage.
B. Acute pulmonary embolism.
C. Arteriovenous malformation.
D. Pulmonary artery aneurysm.

91. A 53-year-old female presents with an approximately 1-year history of worsening shortness of breath. She has a past medical history of diabetes mellitus, hypercholesterolemia, hypertension, and coronary artery disease. She underwent 3-vessel coronary artery bypass grafting 18 months ago. Her postoperative course was complicated by readmission for pleurisy and shortness of breath that was treated as a postpericardotomy syndrome. While her pleurisy resolved, her shortness of breath has progressively worsened. Recently she felt as if she was going to pass out after climbing a flight of steps.

On physical examination vital signs are stable. Examination of the neck veins with the patient lying down at 45° shows prominent a and v wave pulsations. Precordial palpation shows the point of apical impulse to be located left of the midsternum at the 5th interspace. Medial to this a right ventricular thrust is present. Friction fremitus is absent. Auscultation of the heart sounds reveals a normal S1, an accentuated P2, and a right-sided S3. A high-pitched blowing noise that increases with deep inspiration is heard over the right lung. Symmetric pedal edema is present bilaterally.

Chest radiographs show enlargement of both main pulmonary arteries, but there are no pleural effusions or parenchymal densities. Echocardiography demonstrates an increase in right atrial size and also right ventricular hypertrophy. The right ventricular systolic pressure is elevated. Ventilation perfusion scan shows several segmental mismatched defects. Right heart catheterization is performed. The mean pulmonary arterial pressure is 45 mm Hg. Pulmonary capillary wedge pressure is 12 mm Hg. Pulmonary angiography is performed at the same time and shows narrowing of the main pulmonary arteries bilaterally with absence of blood flow to the right lower and left upper pulmonary segments.

Which one of the following should be performed?
A. Pulmonary embolectomy.
B. Thromboendarterectomy.
C. Suction embolectomy.
D. Placement of an inferior vena cava filter and long-term anticoagulation with warfarin.

92. Which one of the following statements about the relationship between obstructive sleep apnea and pulmonary hypertension is true?
A. There is a linear relationship between the severity of the respiratory disturbance index and the severity of pulmonary hypertension.
B. Untreated severe obstructive sleep apnea will eventually lead to sustained pulmonary hypertension and cor pulmonale.
C. Brief repetitive apnea-induced hypoxemia will eventually lead to diurnal pulmonary hypertension.
D. The presence of sustained daytime hypoxemia is a prerequisite for the development of diurnal pulmonary hypertension.

93. A 40-year-old female with a history of asthma, anosmia, and sinusitis is evaluated for worsening respiratory symptoms. She describes the onset of nasal congestion, chest tightness, shortness of breath, cough, and wheezing approximately 1 to 3 hours after exercise. She is training to run a 5-kilometer race. The episodes are occurring more frequently as the race date approaches. A review of symptoms is otherwise unremarkable except for persistent soreness in the quadriceps femoris muscles. Medications include beclomethasone inhaler 40 mcg two inhalations twice daily and an albuterol metered dose inhaler two inhalations 10 minutes before exercise.

Physical examination reveals an athletic-looking female in no distress. Respiratory rate is 16 breaths/min. The lungs are clear to auscultation. Inspection of the thorax reveals no chest wall deformities. There is no evidence of hyperinflation. The expiratory phase is not prolonged. No cardiac murmurs are appreciated. Anterior rhinoscopy shows boggy nasal mucosa bilaterally. Examination of the oropharynx shows minimal cobblestoning. A peak flow performed in the office is not significantly changed from the patient's baseline. A flow volume loop does not suggest any fixed or variable obstruction.

Which one of the following should be advised?
A. Increase albuterol to 4 inhalations, 10 minutes prior to exercise.
B. Begin cromolyn sodium, 4 inhalations 15 to 20 minutes before exercise.
C. Take a further medication history.
D. Advise that the patient not participate in exercise.

94. A 48-year-old female has not felt well for several months. She is experiencing progressive wheezing, cough, and dyspnea with exertion. A review of systems is positive for intermittent vertigo, nasal congestion, mild epistaxis, hoarseness, anterior chest wall discomfort, and pain in the right eye not accompanied by any vision loss. Past medical history is notable for diverticulosis and a prior cholecystectomy. She is not currently on any prescription medications. She denies the use of tobacco products, alcohol, and illicit drugs. She is married with 3 healthy children and works as a bank teller.

Physical examination shows a female in no distress. Temperature is 36.8°C, heart rate is 74 beats/min, blood pressure is 130/82 mm Hg, and respiratory rate is 16 breaths/min. Visual fields are intact. The auricles appear mildly erythematous and are tender to touch. The left sternoclavicular and several costochondral joints are tender to palpation. With the diaphragm of the stethoscope placed over the trachea, a high-pitched noise is heard during inspiration only. Lung sounds are clear. A Westergren erythrocyte sedimentation rate is 62 mm/hr, hematocrit is 38%, leukocyte count is 9,000/cu mm with a normal differential, rheumatoid factor is 1:40, antibodies to double-stranded DNA are 9%, ANA is 1:40, BUN is 12 mg/dL, creatinine is 1.2 mg/dL, serum C3 complement is 198 mg/dL, and C4 complement is 33 mg/dL. Posteroanterior and lateral view chest radiographs suggest tracheal narrowing.

The most likely diagnosis is:
A. Giant cell arteritis.
B. Behcet's disease.
C. Relapsing polychondritis.
D. Rheumatoid arthritis.

95. A 74-year-old female was in her usual state of health until 3 weeks ago. She initially developed what she believed was a minor upper respiratory tract infection with watery eyes, nasal discharge, scratchy throat, fatigue, and a mild nonproductive cough. About a week later, the cough became progressively worse. It can be triggered by the most minor of activities such as talking or laughing. Several times the cough was so violent she thought she might vomit. Her sleep has been disrupted the past couple of nights because of coughing. This morning she became alarmed when she saw a large bright red spot in the corner of her right eye. Past medical history is unremarkable and she is a nonsmoker. She stays home to care for her 6-month-old- great grandson.

On physical examination vital signs are normal. There is a focal, nonraised red area on the lateral ocular surface of the right eye. Auscultation of the lungs reveals no wheezes or crackles. Posteroanterior and lateral view chest radiographs show a normal-size cardiac silhouette and no pleural effusions or parenchymal densities. Leukocyte count is 11,500/cu mm with a normal differential.

Which one of the following interventions should be performed?
A. Prescribe a combination first generation antihistamine with decongestant.
B. Prescribe azithromycin.
C. Prescribe an ipratropium oral inhaler.
D. Prescribe an ipratropium intranasal spray.

96. An 80-year-old male presents with right-sided chest pain, shortness of breath, and a nonproductive cough. Symptoms have been progressive over the last 3 months. A review of systems is positive for fatigue and poor appetite. He has a history of hypertension for which he takes hydrochlorothiazide and obstructive sleep apnea treated with a continuous positive airway pressure device. He is a retired railroad worker. Hobbies include gardening and woodworking. Chest radiographs show a moderate-size right pleural effusion. Pleuroscopy with pleural biopsy is performed. A representative image is shown in figure 96-A. Immunohistochemical staining is positive for calretinin as shown in figure 96-B. Cytokeratin 5/6 staining is also positive.

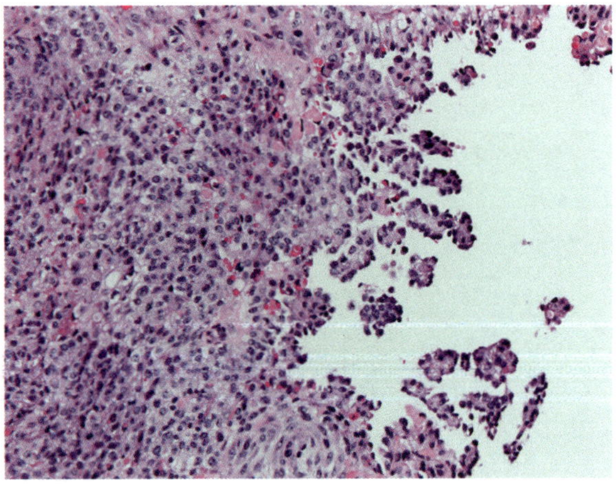

Figure 96-A

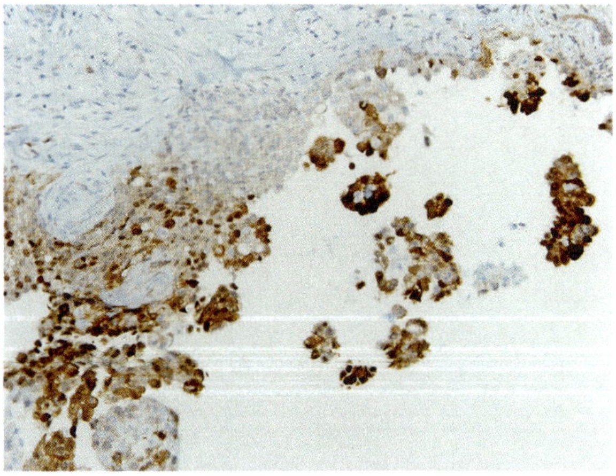

Figure 96-B

Which one of the following statements about this tumor is true?
A. Cigarette smoking is a risk factor.
B. Sarcomatous cell type has a better prognosis than epithelial cell type.
C. Death is usually the result of distant metastatic disease.
D. The tumor originates on the parietal pleura and spreads to the visceral pleura.

97. A 28-year-old female with a history of migraine headaches and epistaxis complains of worsening shortness of breath over the last 6 months. Her condition is aggravated by exertion such as climbing steps. She denies chest pain, dizziness, orthopnea, and paroxysmal nocturnal dyspnea. Her only medication is sumatriptan to use if needed for migraine headache.

On physical examination temperature is 36.7°C, heart rate is 72 beats/min, blood pressure is 119/59 mm Hg, and respiratory rate is 20 breaths/min. With the patient lying supine on the examination table, oxygen saturation measured by pulse oximetery on ambient air is 94%. It decreases to 88% when assuming a standing posture. Cardiopulmonary examination is otherwise unremarkable. There are numerous 2 to 4 mm brown-colored oval lesions scattered across the face, chest, and upper extremities. Examination of the digits of her hand reveals that the angle from the nail bed to the nail is approximately 200°. Leukocyte count is 8,000/cu mm, hematocrit is 37%, hemoglobin is 10 g/dL, MCV is 78 fL, and platelet count is 160,000/cu mm. Computed tomography scanning of the chest following administration of intravenous contrast shows a nodule in the right lower lobe. Representative images are shown in figures 97-A and 97-B.

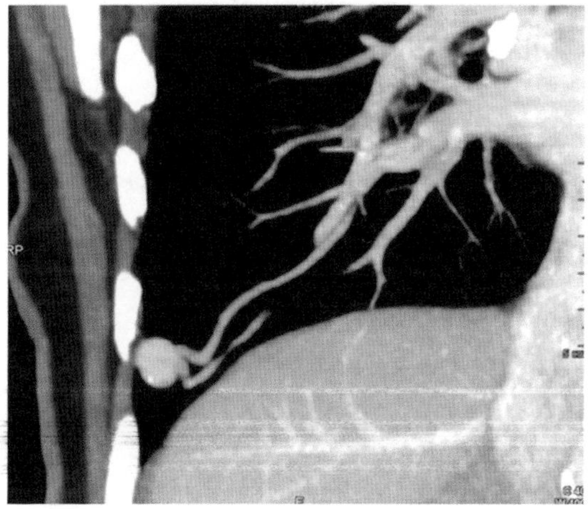

Figure 97-A

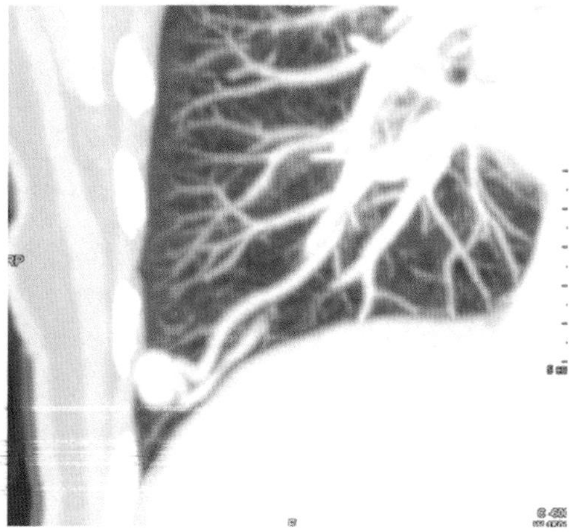

Figure 97-B

Which one of the following should be performed?

A. Administer oral ethinylestradiol and norethisterone.
B. Administer oral tamoxifen.
C. Embolization.
D. Administer intravenous bevacizumab.

98. A 30-year-old female presents with a complaint of cough. She was in her usual state of health until about 10 days ago when she developed a cough productive of greenish sputum. Streaks of bright red blood are occasionally present within the mucus she expectorates. She denies fever, chills, sweats, chest pain, and shortness of breath. She is otherwise healthy and takes no prescription medications. She briefly smoked cigarettes for 6 months while in high school.

On physical examination temperature is 37.1°C, heart rate is 78 beats/min, and respiratory rate is 16 breaths/min. Inspection of the thorax reveals no obvious deformities. Bimanual percussion does not demonstrate any dullness. Vibratory palpation is symmetric without any areas that are increased or diminished. No crackles or wheezes are appreciated with auscultation of the lungs. Whispered and spoken syllables are indistinct.

Which one of the following should be recommended?
A. Doxycycline.
B. $Beta_2$ agonist bronchodilator administered via a metered dose inhaler.
C. Observation.
D. Mucokinetic agent.

99. A 26-year-old female presents to the emergency room following the sudden onset of right-sided chest pain, shortness of breath, and cough. Symptoms developed 30 minutes ago while she was at home watching television. She had a similar episode approximately 1 month ago that was much less severe and gradually resolved over the course of several hours. She did not seek medical attention with that episode. Past medical history is unremarkable except for recurrent low back pain. A review of systems is positive for intermittent abdominal bloating and constipation. She smokes 1 pack of cigarettes a day. She is not on any medications. She denies illicit drug use. On physical examination she is afebrile. Respiratory rate is 24 breaths/min, heart rate 112 beats/min, and blood pressure 154/86mmHg. The trachea is midline. There is hyperresonance with percussion over the right hemithorax along with absent lung sounds and fremitus.

Which one of the following about this condition is true?
A. The majority of pneumothoraces occur on the right side.
B. A chylous pleural effusion is another common manifestation of this condition.
C. High-resolution computed tomography scanning of the chest will show numerous thin-walled cysts bilaterally.
D. Physical examination will reveal numerous skin tags, trichodiscomas, and fibrofolliculomas.

100. A 71-year-old male presents with progressive shortness of breath. He has been symptomatic for the past several months. He denies chest pain, orthopnea, paroxysmal nocturnal dyspnea, and cough. A review of systems is positive for fatigue, anorexia, and cachexia. He has a history of alcoholism.

On physical examination the patient is afebrile. He appears alert and oriented. Cardiac examination reveals a normal S1 and S2 without any gallop or murmur. Lung sounds are clear to auscultation. Palmer erythema is evident. He has engorged superficial veins on the upper abdomen. Spider nevi are present on the thorax. Gynecomastia is noted bilaterally. There is pitting edema of the lower extremities bilaterally. Testicular atrophy is present. The liver edge is palpable, but appears firm and nontender. Arterial blood gas performed on ambient air shows a pH of 7.45, $PaCO_2$ of 36 mm Hg, and a PaO_2 of 60 mm Hg. A contrast enhanced transesophageal echocardiogram is performed following administration of saline in a peripheral vein. Numerous microbubbles are appreciated in the left atrium within four cardiac cycles.

Which one of the following should be recommended?

A. Inhaled nitric oxide.
B. Oral propanolol.
C. Liver transplantation.
D. Transjugular intrahepatic portosystemic shunt.

ANSWERS

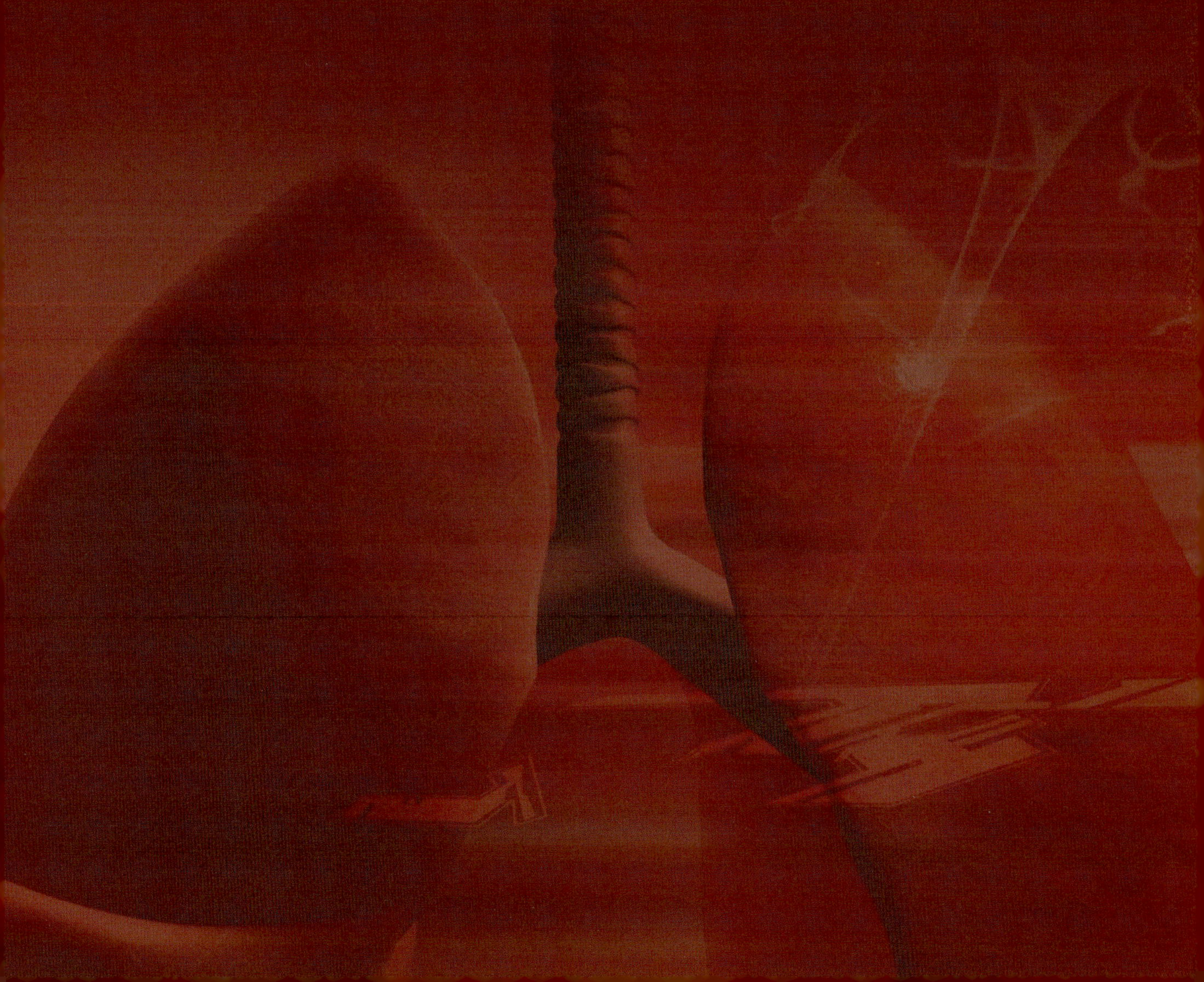

1. C. A single transbronchial biopsy reveals granulomatous inflammation with acid-fast bacilli present.

SUBJECT: Nontuberculous mycobacterial lung disease

The most common nontuberculous mycobacteria causing chronic pulmonary disease are species of the mycobacterium avium complex (*M. avium* and *M. intracellulare*) and *M. kansasii*. The classic patient with a mycobacterium avium complex infection is a postmenopausal female who is thin. Other physical features described include scoliosis, pectus excavatum, and mitral valve prolapse. Presenting symptoms are usually cough, fatigue, and malaise. Dyspnea, fever, hemoptysis, and weight loss are sometimes present. Imaging findings are variable but include tiny nodules, infiltrates, bronchiectasis, and cavities.

Criteria for diagnosis include the proper clinical presentation and supportive microbiologic data. Below are the acceptable microbiologic criteria.

1. Positive culture from at least 2 separate expectorated sputa samples, or
2. Positive culture results from at least 1 bronchial wash or lavage, or
3. Lung biopsy with mycobacterial histopathologic features (granulomatous inflammation or the presence of acid-fast bacilli) and a positive culture, or
4. Lung biopsy with mycobacterial histopathologic features (granulomatous inflammation or the presence of acid-fast bacilli) and1 or more sputum/bronchial washing that is culture positive.

Answers A, B, and D all satisfy the criteria for a diagnosis. Answer C does not. Although the biopsy shows mycobacterial histopathologic features, a positive culture of the organism is lacking.

Griffith DE, Aksamit T, Brown-Elliott BA, et al. An official ATS/IDSA statement: Diagnosis, treatment, and prevention of nontuberculous mycobacterial disease. *Am J Respir Crit Care Med* 2007; 175:367-416.

2. D. Individuals may return to the workplace/environment and be re-exposed to low levels of the causative agent without becoming symptomatic.

SUBJECT: Reactive airways dysfunction syndrome

Reactive airway dysfunction syndrome (RADS) is a type of irritant-induced asthma. Features of RADS include the following:

- Documented absence of preceding respiratory symptoms.
- Onset of symptoms after a single exposure incident.

- Symptoms correlate with exposure to a toxic substance such as a gas, smoke, fume, or vapor in very high concentrations (answer A is incorrect).
- Onset of symptoms usually within minutes to hours, and always within 24 hours, with persistence of symptoms for at least 3 months (answer C is incorrect).
- Symptoms simulate asthma.
- Presence of airflow obstruction and/or presence of nonspecific bronchial hyperresponsiveness with pulmonary function testing.
- Other pulmonary diseases are excluded.

The treatment of RADS is similar to the treatment of asthma. Re-exposure to the toxic substance at low concentrations is considered safe. Individuals with RADS may, therefore, return to the workplace/ environment associated with the causative agent if measures are taken to limit exposure thresholds.

Atopy is not a risk factor for the development of RADS (answer B is incorrect).

Alberts WM, do Pico GA. Reactive airways dysfunction syndrome. *Chest* 1996; 109:1618-1626.

3. A. Malignant transformation is uncommon.

<u>SUBJECT</u>: Lymphoid interstitial pneumonia

Lymphoid interstitial pneumonia (LIP) is characterized by a dense interstitial infiltrate comprised mostly of T-lymphocytes (answer B is incorrect), plasma cells, and macrophages (figures 3-B and 3-C.

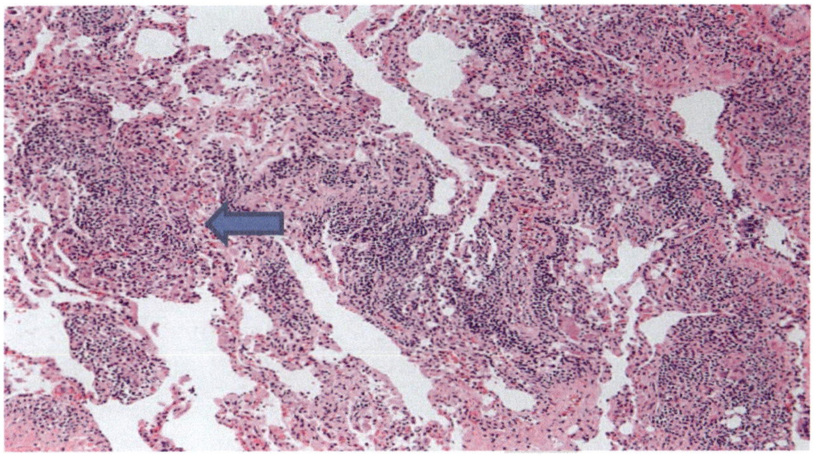

Figure 3-B

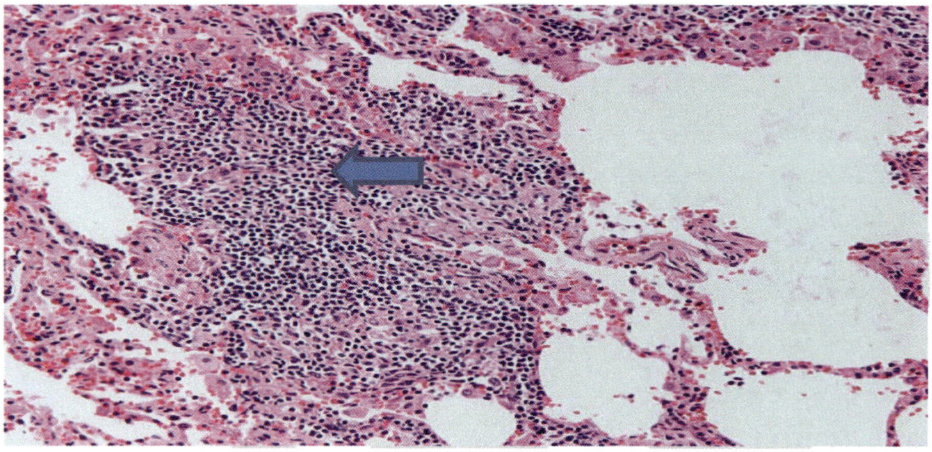

Figure 3-C

The arrows point to an area of dense T-lymphocyte infiltration). Lymphoid hyperplasia may be present. Organizing pneumonia and necrotizing granulomas are absent. The histologic differential diagnosis includes hyperplasia of bronchial mucosa-associated lymphoid tissue and lymphoma. It was once believed that most cases of LIP would develop into lymphoma, but it is now recognized that only a small number of cases actually undergo a malignant transformation.

LIP has been described in the setting of several disorders such as Sjögren's syndrome (which the patient in this question has), Hashimoto's disease, systemic lupus erythematosus, primary biliary cirrhosis, and rheumatoid arthritis. The incidence of idiopathic LIP is thought to be low.

Diagnosis of LIP typically requires a surgical biopsy. Immunohistochemistry and molecular analysis can usually differentiate LIP from a lymphoproliferative disorder. Clonality should not be present in LIP (answer C is incorrect). The finding of lymphocytosis in the bronchoalveolar lavage fluid is not diagnostic of LIP. The natural history of LIP is poorly understood. There are no clinical trials that have defined the optimal approach to therapy. Some cases will stabilize without any treatment. There are reports of patients having a dramatic response or complete remission with glucocorticoid therapy. While progression to end-stage fibrosis and death sometimes occurs, it is not inevitable in all cases (answer D is incorrect).

American Thoracic Society. American Thoracic Society/European Respiratory Society international multidisciplinary consensus classification of the idiopathic interstitial pneumonias. *Am J Respir Crit Care Med* 2002; 165:277-304.

4. A. Enroll in hospice.

<u>SUBJECT</u>: Hospice care

Any patient who is in the terminal phase of a pulmonary disease (life expectancy of 6 months or less) may benefit from enrollment in hospice. Criteria for eligibility include severe chronic lung disease with disabling dyspnea at rest, lack of response to bronchodilators, fatigue, postbronchodilator FEV_1 less than 30% of predicted, and progression of end-stage pulmonary disease characterized by increasing visits to the emergency room or hospitalization. Additional criteria include hypoxemia at rest ($PaO_2 \leq 55$ mm Hg on ambient air or oxygen saturation $\leq 88\%$ on supplemental oxygen), hypercapnia with a $PaCO_2 > 50$ mm Hg, the presence of cor pulmonale, unintentional progressive weight loss (> 10% of body weight over the preceding 6 months), and resting tachycardia > 100 beats/min.

Replacement therapy with alpha-1 antiprotease is not recommended for individuals who have heterozygous phenotypes and a normal alpha-1 antitrypsin plasma level (answer B is incorrect). The patient in this question has several contraindications to lung volume reduction surgery including active cigarette smoking, homogeneous distribution of emphysema, and significant co-morbid conditions that increase the risk for surgical mortality (answer C is incorrect). Lung transplantation is also contraindicated because of smoking status and other vital organ dysfunction (answer D is incorrect).

Lanken PN, Terry PB, DeLisser HM, et al. An official American Thoracic Society clinical policy statement: Palliative care for patients with respiratory diseases and critical illnesses. *Am J Respir Crit Care Med* 2008; 177:912-927.

5. D. Systemic hypotension.

<u>SUBJECT</u>: Pulmonary embolism and thrombolytic therapy

The patient in this question has an acute pulmonary embolism (PE). A pleural rub is evident on physical examination. The use of thrombolytics for the treatment of acute PE remains controversial, and there are no definitive data confirming a reduction in mortality. The decision to use thrombolytics must be determined on a case-by-case basis. The only widely accepted indication is systemic hypotension, defined as a systolic blood pressure < 90 mm Hg.

Potential indications for the administration of systemic thrombolytic include: severe, refractory hypoxemia (answer C is incorrect), patent foramen ovale, and right atrial or ventricular thrombus. The presence of right ventricular dysfunction on echocardiography is a predictor of mortality and is therefore considered a potential indication for thrombolytic administration. A finding of severe pulmonary hypertension on echocardiography is not an established indication (answer A is incorrect). The size of a perfusion defect on ventilation-perfusion scanning is also not an established indication (answer C is incorrect). It is recommended that thrombolytic therapy be administered using a short infusion time (2 hours) over a more prolonged infusion time. The agent should be administered into a peripheral vein instead of through a pulmonary artery catheter.

Relative contraindications for administering thrombolytic therapy include uncontrolled hypertension, cerebrovascular accident within the last 2 months, platelet count < 100,000/cu mm, and surgery within the last 10 days. Absolute contraindications to thrombolytic therapy include intracranial neoplasm, history of hemorrhagic stroke, intracranial surgery within the past 2 months, major trauma, active bleeding, and significant internal bleeding within the last 6 months.

Kearon C, Akl E, Comerota A, et al. Antithrombotic therapy for VTE disease: Antithrombotic therapy and prevention of thrombosis, 9th ed: American College of Chest Physicians evidence-based clinical practice guidelines. *Chest* 2012; 141 (2) (Suppl):e419S-e494S.

6. A. Thoracotomy with surgical resection.

SUBJECT: Bronchogenic cyst

A bronchogenic cyst is a common bronchopulmonary malformation. It is a result of an abnormal budding of the tracheobronchial tree separate from the primary airway. It is most commonly located in the mediastinum although it can also be intraparenchymal. Rare cases have also described bronchogenic cysts in the diaphragm, pericardium, neck, and abdomen. The cyst wall is lined with ciliated pseudostratified columnar epithelium and may contain bronchial mucous glands, cartilage, and smooth muscle. The differential diagnosis of a bronchogenic cyst includes lymphoma, teratoma, metastatic cancer, and lymphadenopathy

Chest radiographs usually demonstrate a rounded, well-demarcated, noncalcified mass. Computed tomography scanning will show a sharply marginated, smooth-walled, well-demarcated, homogenous, low-attenuation (0-20 Hounsfield units) mass without vascular enhancement.

Many bronchogenic cysts are found incidentally in asymptomatic patients. Nevertheless, surgical resection, either with a traditional thoracotomy or thorascopically with video assistance, is recommended, as the majority of cysts will eventually become symptomatic. The most common presenting symptoms include cough and chest pain. Other reported complications include compression of mediastinal structures, infection, hemoptysis, and hemorrhage within the cyst. Malignancy arising from a cyst has also been documented.

Fine needle aspiration of a cyst is not recommended as the definitive therapeutic intervention given the high likelihood of cyst recurrence in the future (answers B and C are incorrect). Because even asymptomatic cysts can potentially become symptomatic and be associated with serious complications, observation in surgical candidates is not appropriate (answer D is incorrect).

Patel SR, Meeker DP, Biscotti CV, et al. Presentation and management of bronchogenic cysts in the adult. *Chest* 1994; 106:79-85.

7. B. There is an increase in minute ventilation as a result of an increase in tidal volume.

SUBJECT: Pregnancy and respiratory physiology

Minute ventilation increases by 20% to 50% before the end of the 1st trimester during normal pregnancy (answer D is incorrect). It remains elevated for the duration of the pregnancy. The rise in minute ventilation is due to a 40% increase in tidal volume (450-600 ml). There is no significant change in the respiratory rate (answers A and C are incorrect). There is an elevation in the progesterone level beginning at 6 weeks of pregnancy that continues through the 37th week. This hormone is responsible for the increase in minute ventilation. Because of the chronic hyperventilation, a normal $PaCO_2$ during pregnancy is 28-32 mm Hg.

Elkus R, Popovich J. Respiratory physiology in pregnancy. *Clin Chest Med* 1992; 13:555-565.

8. B. Skin biopsy will show tight, well-formed caseating granulomas.

SUBJECT: Sarcoidosis

Sarcoidosis is a multisystem disorder of uncertain etiology. It tends to occur in adults less than 40 years old. In the United States, it is more common in blacks than whites. Almost every organ system can be affected, with lung involvement present in more than 90% of patients. The hallmark of sarcoidosis is the characteristic lesion of a noncaseating granuloma. The granuloma is usually well formed and surrounded by a rim of lymphocytes and fibroblasts.

Löfgren's syndrome, which the patient in this question has, refers to a variant of sarcoidosis characterized by fever, erythema nodosum, and arthralgias. Chest radiographs will show bilateral hilar lymphadenopathy. Less common symptoms include facial (Bell's) palsy and iritis (answer C is a true statement). At the time of presentation the angiotensin converting enzyme level is characteristically normal in the majority of individuals (answer D is a true statement). Histological examination of an erythema nodosum lesion will not show the characteristic granuloma of sarcoidosis. Rather, there will be nonspecific findings of panniculitis, without evidence of vasculitis.

The prognosis of Löfgren's syndrome is generally excellent. The condition usually spontaneously resolves (answer A is a true statement). Fever and erythema nodosum typically resolve within weeks, other manifestations such as adenopathy may take longer.

American Thoracic Society. Statement on sarcoidosis. *Am J Respir Crit Care Med* 1999; 160:736-755.

9. D. Prednisone and itraconazole.

SUBJECT: Allergic bronchopulmonary aspergillosis

Allergic bronchopulmonary aspergillosis (ABPA) is caused by a hypersensitivity reaction to *Aspergillus fumigatus* that colonize the bronchi. The prevalence is approximately 1% to 2% in patients with asthma and 2% to 15% in patients with cystic fibrosis. The majority of patients will present with respiratory symptoms of wheezing, bronchial hyperreactivity, and cough. It is common to expectorate brown mucus plugs. Hemoptysis and a low-grade fever may also be present. Physical examination may be normal, but expiratory wheezes are commonly present. Digital clubbing is seen in approximately 15% of patients. Characteristic imaging findings include multilobar bronchiectasis, mucoid impaction, mosaic attenuation, tree-in-bud opacities, and centrilobular nodules.

The major criteria for the diagnosis of ABPA are:

- Asthma.
- Roentgenographic fleeting pulmonary infiltrates.
- Central bronchiectasis.
- Peripheral blood eosinophilia.
- Precipitating antibodies (IgG) to *A. fumigatus.*
- Increased serum total IgE (> 1,000 IU/mL).

- *A. fumigatus* specific IgG and IgE.
- A positive skin reaction to Aspergillus antigen.

The stages of ABPA are:
I. Acute phase.
II. Remission.
III. Exacerbation.
IV. Glucocorticoid dependent.
V. End stage (fibrotic).

Oral glucocorticoids are the treatment of choice for ABPA. The addition of itraconazole allows for a reduction in the dose of glucocorticoids and leads to fewer exacerbations. Therefore consideration should be given to using this antifungal agent along with glucocorticoids after the first relapse of ABPA or in patients with glucocorticoid dependent ABPA. Monotherapy with an antifungal agent would not be adequate treatment (answer B is incorrect). Omalizumab is a monoclonal antibody directed against IgE. Although there is interest in the use of this agent in cystic fibrosis patients with ABPA, use is not currently recommended pending more definitive studies (answer A is incorrect). There is no established role for use of inhaled glucocorticoids in the treatment of ABPA (answer C is incorrect).

Agarwal, R. Allergic bronchopulmonary aspergillosis. *Chest* 2009; 135:805-826.

10. B. Increase in survival.

SUBJECT: Pulmonary rehabilitation

Pulmonary rehabilitation is an evidence-based, multidisciplinary program for patients with chronic respiratory diseases. For individuals with chronic obstructive pulmonary disease, a number of benefits have been demonstrated, including an improvement in the symptom of dyspnea (answer A is a true statement), improvement in health-related quality of life, a reduction in the number of hospital days for acute exacerbations (answer C is a true statement), and other measures of health care utilization (answer D is a true statement), as well as psychosocial benefits. To date, there is insufficient evidence to conclude that it improves survival.

Ries AL, Bauldoff GS, Casaburi R, et al. Pulmonary rehabilitation: Joint ACCP/AACVPR evidence-based clinical practice guidelines. *Chest* 2007; 131:4S-42S.

11. A. Normal expiratory reserve volume.

SUBJECT: Obesity and pulmonary function testing

The World Health Organization defines obesity as a body mass index >30 kg/m^2. The increased weight against the chest wall changes respiratory mechanics and results in a decrease in compliance. Obesity typically does not result in a change in the FEV_1 or FVC. The ratio should therefore be normal (answer C is a true statement). The maximal voluntary ventilation may be decreased, possibly because the diaphragm is at a mechanical disadvantage due to being displaced into the thoracic cavity because of abdominal girth. With respect to lung volumes, the functional residual capacity and expiratory reserve volume are reduced. The expiratory reserve volume is reduced greater than the functional residual capacity with increasing obesity. The residual volume and total lung capacity are typically normal (answer B is a true statement). The diffusion capacity is also typically preserved (answer D is a true statement).

With extreme obesity a decrease in the FEV_1, FVC, and total lung capacity can be seen. For these changes to occur the BMI is usually ~ 45 kg/m^2 or greater.

Unterborn J. Pulmonary function testing in obesity, pregnancy, and extremes of body habitus. *Clin Chest Med* 2001; 22:759-767.

12. D. Despite drug withdrawal, the majority of patients will have residual chronic fibrosis.

SUBJECT: Methotrexate-induced pulmonary toxicity

Methotrexate is a folic acid antagonist. It is used in the treatment of a variety of conditions, including rheumatoid arthritis, inflammatory bowel disease, and psoriasis. Methotrexate-induced pulmonary toxicity has a prevalence of approximately 1% to 8%. A number of conditions have been described, including inflammatory disorders (hypersensitivity pneumonitis, organizing pneumonia, diffuse alveolar damage, pleural effusion), opportunistic infections, and pulmonary lymphoproliferative disorders.

Methotrexate-induced hypersensitivity pneumonitis typically occurs days to months after initiating therapy. Fever, shortness of breath, cough, arthralgias, and rash may be seen (answer A is a true statement). Mediastinal and hilar lymphadenopathy occur in approximately 10% to 15% of patients (answer C is a true statement). Nearly half of patients will have a peripheral eosinophilia (answer B is a true statement). With drug withdrawal, the prognosis is generally favorable, and less than 10% of patients will develop chronic fibrosis.

Treatment of methotrexate-induced hypersensitivity pneumonitis consists of drug withdrawal. If there is a concern that infection is present, bronchoscopy with bronchoalveolar lavage should be performed. Biopsy is generally not required and should be reserved for patients whose course is complicated. Treatment with glucocorticoids remains controversial. Administration may accelerate recovery in some cases.

Imokawa S, Colby TV, Leslie KO, et al. Methotrexate pneumonitis: review of the literature and histopathological findings in nine patients. *Eur Respir J* 2000; 15:373-381.

13. B. The majority of cases occur in cigarette smokers.

SUBJECT: Desquamative interstitial pneumonitis

Desquamative interstitial pneumonitis (DIP) is one of the idiopathic interstitial pneumonias. It was originally thought that this condition was characterized by desquamation of epithelial cells, but it is now recognized that this is not true. The disorder is characterized by intra-alveolar macrophage accumulation. DIP occurs almost exclusively in cigarette smokers. It is more common in men than women (answer C is incorrect). Disease onset is usually in the 4th or 5th decade. The condition is characterized by the subacute onset of dyspnea and dry cough and may progress to fulminate respiratory failure. With smoking cessation, the prognosis is generally good. Many cases seem to respond to the administration of glucocorticoids. The prognosis is better than that observed with usual interstitial pneumonitis (answer A is incorrect).

Pulmonary function test usually shows normal lung volumes or mild restriction with a decreased diffusion capacity. Chest radiographic findings are nonspecific and may even be normal. Computed tomography findings include ground glass opacities with a lower zone distribution. The opacities are usually diffuse, uniform, and peripheral. Honeycombing is seen in under a third of cases (answer D is incorrect). Bronchoalveolar lavage may show increased alveolar macrophages with "smoker's pigment," which consists of intracellular yellow, brown, or black smoke particulates. Video-assisted thorascopic lung biopsy is usually required for diagnosis. Characteristic histologic features include homogeneous involvement of lung parenchyma, accumulation of alveolar macrophages, mild/moderate thickening of alveolar septa, and interstitial inflammation (figure 13-C). Findings of extensive fibrosis, smooth muscle proliferation, eosinophils, and organizing pneumonia should be inconspicuous or absent.

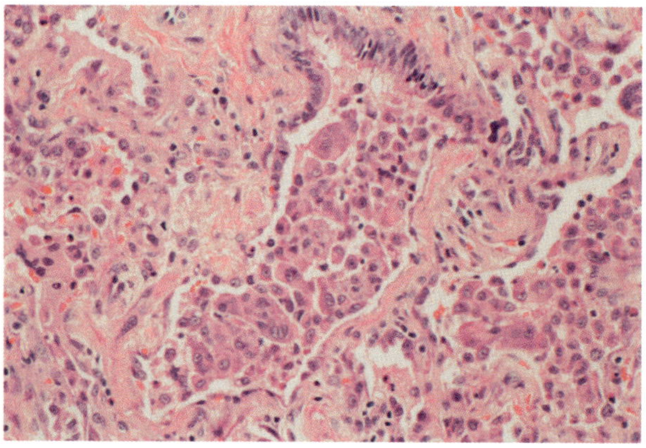

Figure 13-C

American Thoracic Society. American Thoracic Society/European Respiratory Society international multidisciplinary consensus classification of the idiopathic interstitial pneumonias. *Am J Respir Crit Care Med* 2002; 165:277-304.

14. D. Streptomycin.

SUBJECT: Pneumonic tularemia

Francisella tularensis is a gram-negative coccobacillus that causes tularemia, a zoonotic infection that occurs primarily in the Northern Hemisphere. There have been 2 outbreaks of pneumonic tularemia at Martha's Vineyard, one in the summer of 1978 and a second in the year 2000. The organism can be transmitted in a number of ways. Many animals such as rabbits, hares, squirrels, muskrats, mice, and beavers can harbor *F. tularensis*. Skinning or eating infected animals are the primary modes of transmission. The organism can also be transmitted through scratches or bites from infected animals. Arthropods can serve as a vector for transmission. A number of tick species, including the wood tick, have been shown to carry *F. tularensis*. Finally, it is believed that *F. tularensis* can become aerosolized, which may explain how activities such as farming and landscaping can be risk factors for infection.

Pneumonic tularemia can result from either inhalation of contaminated material or from hematogenous spread. Symptoms include abrupt onset fever and headache followed by nonproductive cough, chest pain, and shortness of breath. A number of different radiographic features have been described including nodular infiltrates, adenopathy, pleural effusion, and less commonly cavitary lesions or a miliary pattern. Making a diagnosis can be a challenge because the organism is difficult to grow with standard culture media. A 4-fold rise in antibody levels between acute and convalescent titers, an acute agglutination titer of 1:160, or an acute microagglutination of 1:128 is considered presumptive of infection.

First line therapy for treatment of moderate to severe pneumonic tularemia is an aminoglycoside. Streptomycin has a well-established efficacy and remains the drug of choice. Gentamicin is an effective alternative. Seven to ten days of therapy is considered adequate. For mild disease, appropriate antimicrobial agents include tetracyclines and ciprofloxacin. Daptomycin, vancomycin, and ceftriaxone are not active against *F. tularensis* (answers A, B, and C are incorrect).

Thomas LD, Schaffner W. Tularemia pneumonia. *Infect Dis Clin N Am* 2010; 24:43-55.

15. B. Insert a 12 Fr catheter attached to a water seal device followed by admission to the hospital.

SUBJECT: Pneumothorax

A spontaneous pneumothorax can be classified as primary (absence of any underlying lung disease) or secondary (in the setting of underlying lung disease). The most common cause of a primary spontaneous pneumothorax is rupture of a subpleural bleb. Risk factors include smoking, body habitus (more common in taller and thinner individuals), and age between early 20s and late 30s. Common presenting symptoms are dyspnea and chest pain. A pneumothorax is considered small in size if it measures less than 3 cm from the apex to cupola. Greater than 3 cm is considered a large pneumothorax. A patient would be considered stable if the respiratory rate is less than 24 breaths/min, heart rate is between 60 and 120 beats/min, blood pressure is normotensive, and there is no hypoxia.

A patient with a small pneumothorax who is stable can be managed with observation alone. If there is no worsening of the radiographic findings or clinical status after 3-6 hours, discharge with follow-up in 12 hours to 2 days is appropriate. A patient with a large pneumothorax, even if stable, should be admitted to the hospital for management (answer A is incorrect). The patient should undergo a procedure to re-expand the lung. This may be accomplished by using either a small-bore catheter (< 14 Fr) or placement of a 16-22 Fr chest tube (answer C is incorrect). The catheter or tube can then be attached to either a water seal device or a Heimlich valve. Suction should be applied if the lung fails to re-expand. Once there is resolution of the pneumothorax, the catheter or chest tube can be removed. For clinically unstable patients with a large pneumothorax, insertion of a 16-22 Fr chest tube should be performed. A larger chest tube may be inserted if it is anticipated that the patient may have a prolonged air leak. The chest tube should be attached to a water seal device and suction applied if necessary.

It is not necessary to perform a procedure to prevent the recurrence of a primary spontaneous pneumothorax unless the initial course is complicated by a nonresolving air leak (answer D is incorrect). An exception to this approach might be if the patient participates in activities such as flying or scuba diving where the risk of recurrent pneumothorax would be potentially serious. Patients undergoing surgical intervention should have a bullectomy performed if apical bullae are visualized. Intraoperative pleurodesis should also be simultaneously performed.

Baumann MH, Strange C, Heffner JE, et al. Management of spontaneous pneumothorax. *Chest* 2001; 119:590-602.

16. C. Creatinine clearance of 46 mg/ml/min.

<u>**SUBJECT**</u>: Lung transplantation

The following conditions are considered relative contraindications to lung transplantation:
- Symptomatic osteoporosis.
- Severe musculoskeletal disease.
- Current use of corticosteroids.
- Requirement for invasive ventilation.
- Colonization with fungi or atypical mycobacteria.
- Adequately treated *Mycobacterium tuberculosis*.
- A documented history of noncompliance with medical care.

Absolute contraindications to lung transplantation include:
- Progressive neuromuscular disease.
- Ideal body weight < 70% or > 130%.
- Substance addiction within the last 6 months.
- Unresolvable psychosocial problems.
- Dysfunction in major organs other than the lung (particularly renal dysfunction defined as a creatinine clearance of < 50 mg/ml/min.).
- Infection with the human immunodeficiency virus.
- Hepatitis B antigen positivity.
- History of hepatitis C with biopsy proven evidence of liver disease.
- Active malignancy within the last 2 years (excluding squamous cell and basal cell carcinoma of the skin).
- Individuals with level > 3 melanoma, colon cancer staged > Dukes A, extra capsular renal cell tumors, and breast cancer > stage 2 within the last 5 years.
- Age > 55 for heart/lung transplants, age > 65 for single lung transplants, and age > 60 for bilateral lung transplants.

American Thoracic Society. International guidelines for the selection of lung transplant candidates. *Am Respir Crit Care Med* 1998; 158:335-339.

17. A. Prednisone.

<u>**SUBJECT**</u>**:** Allergic angiitis and granulomatosis

Allergic angiitis and granulomatosis (formerly known as Churg-Strauss syndrome) is a systemic disorder characterized predominantly by rhinitis, asthma, and peripheral eosinophilia. The classic case progresses through 3 distinct phases: prodromal phase characterized by atopic diseases, eosinophilic phase characterized by peripheral eosinophilia with infiltration of various organs, and a systemic vasculitis phase. This usually develops 8-10 years after the onset of atopic disease. The mean age of onset of the vasculitis phase is approximately 38. Men and women are equally affected.

Allergic angiitis and granulomatosis can involve nearly every organ system. Upper airway manifestations include sinusitis, rhinitis, and nasal polyps. Cutaneous findings include palpable purpura and urticaria. Neurologic manifestations include mononeuritis multiplex, which can present as "wrist drop" and "foot drop." Nerve infarction can lead to muscle atrophy. Pulmonary findings include migratory pulmonary infiltrates. Pleural effusions are seen in the minority of cases. Additional manifestations include eosinophilic gastroenteritis, pericarditis, heart failure, renal insufficiency, and generalized lymphadenopathy.

When lung biopsy is performed, the pathology demonstrates necrotizing giant cell vasculitis, predominantly involving the small arteries. Granulomas are frequently present, as are extravascular eosinophils. Transbronchial biopsy is usually insufficient to make a diagnosis.

A number of laboratory abnormalities have been described. Marked eosinophilia is typically present (usually greater than 10% of the total leukocyte count). Other commonly observed abnormalities include a normochromic, normocytic anemia, elevated IgE, positive rheumatoid factor, and normal complement levels. Approximately 50% of the patients will have a positive ANCA. Antibodies directed against proteinase 3 (C-ANCA) and against myeloperoxidase (P-ANCA) have been described with the latter being more common.

The primary treatment is glucocorticoids. Institution of prednisone usually results in a complete remission in the majority of patients, even those with multisystem organ involvement. Even in patients who achieve a successful remission, long-term low-dose prednisone therapy is usually required. Untreated disease has a high mortality rate with approximately 50% dying in the first 3 months following the onset of vasculitis. Cyclophosphamide has been administered in some cases in combination with glucocorticoids. There are not substantial data to support other treatments such as intravenous immunoglobulin therapy or plasma exchange (answers B, C, and D are incorrect).

Allen, JN, Davis WB. Eosinophilic lung diseases. *Am J Respir Crit Care Med* 1994; 150:1423-1438.

18. A. Pulmonary function testing will be normal.

SUBJECT: Kyphoscoliosis and respiratory mechanics

Kyphoscoliosis can be congenital, idiopathic, or secondary. Most cases that are idiopathic present during late adolescence or early adulthood. Secondary cases can occur in association with a number of conditions such as muscular dystrophy, cerebral palsy, or prior thoracoplasty. Kyphoscoliosis has a characteristic anterior/posterior angulation of the spine. Radiographs can be used to measure the degree of spinal deformity (Cobb angle). Patients with mild kyphoscoliosis (Cobb angles $< 25^{\circ}$) usually have normal pulmonary function, normal gas exchange, and exercise capacity with a favorable prognosis. Moderate kyphoscoliosis (Cobb angles 25° to 75°) is usually associated with reduced exercise capacity and nocturnal oxyhemoglobin desaturation. A restrictive ventilatory defect is evident with angles $> 90^{\circ}$. Severe kyphoscoliosis (angles $> 100^{\circ}$) is usually accompanied by significant respiratory symptoms and risk for respiratory failure. Because the individual in this example has a Cobb angle of 20°, answers B, C, and D are incorrect.

Indications for long-term noninvasive positive pressure ventilation for chest wall disorders includes the following: chronic respiratory failure with a daytime arterial $PaCO_2 \geq 45$ mm Hg, evidence of nocturnal oxyhemoglobin desaturation less than 88% for > 5 consecutive minutes or > 10% of the total sleep time, cor pulmonale, hypersomnolence, dyspnea, morning headaches, and fatigue.

Tzelepis,G, McCool, FD. The lungs and chest wall diseases. In: Textbook of Respiratory Medicine 5th Edition, Murray, JF, Nadel, JA (Eds), Saunders Elsevier, Philadelphia 2010.

19. B. Coexistent asthma is common.

SUBJECT: Chronic eosinophilic pneumonia

The cause of chronic eosinophilic pneumonia (CEP) remains unknown. It occurs more commonly in females than males (2:1) with the peak incidence in the 5th decade. The onset is subacute with many patients having symptoms about 8 months before diagnosis. Cough, fever, dyspnea, and weight loss are typical symptoms. Asthma is present in approximately 50% of cases, oftentimes for several years prior to the diagnosis. A peripheral blood eosinophilia is present in close to 90% of patients. A serum IgE level is increased in about two-thirds of patients. The chest radiograph finding of dense, extensive, bilateral, peripheral infiltrates (the so-called "photographic negative pulmonary edema") is present in approximately 25% of patients (answer A is incorrect). Similar radiographic changes have also been described in organizing pneumonia, sarcoidosis, and drug reactions.

Lung biopsy is not required for diagnosis (answer C is incorrect). Bronchoalveolar lavage can easily detect the presence of alveolar eosinophilia (figure 19-A. The arrow points to an eosinophil). During the acute stage of CEP, the eosinophil count is in excess of 25%. This finding is supportive of a diagnosis provided other causes of pulmonary eosinophilia have been excluded. The differential diagnosis of lavage eosinophilia > 25% includes allergic angiitis and granulomatosis, drug-induced pneumonitis, and parasitic infection. The great majority of patients require treatment with prednisone, with fewer than 10% having a spontaneous resolution. Most patients will have a relapse of symptoms if prednisone is discontinued within the first 6 months of treatment. These patients will require a slower taper. A minority of patients will require treatment indefinitely (answer D is incorrect).

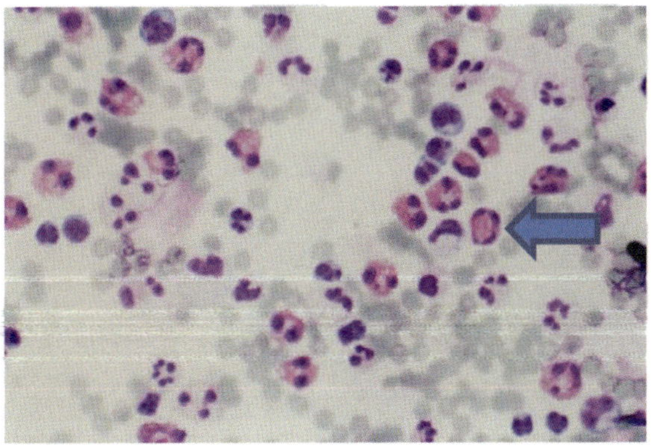

Figure 19-A

Allen, JN, Davis WB. Eosinophilic lung diseases. *Am J Respir Crit Care Med* 1994; 150:1423-1438.

20. B. The patient is likely a current or former cigarette smoker.

SUBJECT: Human immunodeficiency virus associated bronchogenic carcinoma

Individuals with HIV are at an increased risk for lung cancer. The most common cell type is adenocarcinoma followed by squamous cell carcinoma. The patient in this question has invasive adenocarcinoma, acinar predominant. Epidemiologic studies indicate most individuals are current or former cigarette smokers. There are some data that suggest HIV infection may be an independent risk factor for lung cancer. The incidence of lung cancer has not decreased in the era of antiretroviral therapy (answer D is incorrect). There does not appear to be any relationship between the CD4 T-cell count, plasma viral levels, and the risk for malignancy. Herpes simplex virus-8 plays an oncogenic role in Kaposi's sarcoma but has not been implicated as a risk factor for bronchogenic carcinoma (answer C is incorrect).

The presentation of lung cancer in HIV-infected individuals mimics that of noninfected individuals. Diagnosis and treatment are also similar. Median survival is similar to age-match HIV-uninfected lung cancer patients (answer A is incorrect).

Morris A, Crothers K, Beck JM, et al. An official ATS workshop report: Emerging issues and current controversies in HIV-associated pulmonary diseases. *Proc Am Thorac Soc* 2011; 8:17-26.

21. B. Provide reassurance and supportive care.

SUBJECT: Vocal cord dysfunction

Vocal cord dysfunction refers to the airway obstruction that occurs with inappropriate movement of the vocal cords. With normal inspiration true vocal cords abduct. With paradoxical vocal cord motion, there is adduction. This can occur with inspiration, expiration, or during both. Conditions associated with vocal cord dysfunction include psychogenic disorders, gastroesophageal reflux, rhinosinusitis, exercise, olfactory stimuli, and chemical irritants. Use of cleaning products containing the chemical irritant ammonia triggered this patient's illness. The differential diagnosis of vocal cord dysfunction includes paroxysmal laryngospasm, laryngeal angioedema, vocal cord paresis/paralysis, and supraglottic disorders.

Vocal cord dysfunction is commonly mistaken for asthma. Typical symptoms of vocal cord dysfunction include throat tightness, a choking sensation, dysphonia, cough, and stridor. An acute event may escalate into respiratory distress. During such an episode, the primary treatment is reassurance and supportive care. There may be a role for inhalation of a helium-oxygen mixture or noninvasive positive pressure ventilation in some cases. Endotracheal intubation is not indicated (answer A is incorrect). Beta agonists, magnesium, and glucocorticoids have not been shown to be beneficial (answers C and D are incorrect).

Visualization of the vocal cords with direct fiberoptic laryngoscopy during an acute attack allows a confident diagnosis to be made. The classic finding is inspiratory vocal cord adduction of the anterior two-thirds with a posterior chink. If performed, a flow volume loop may show truncation of the inspiratory limb consistent with a variable extrathoracic obstruction. Pulmonary function testing should be normal between attacks.

Morris MJ, Christopher KL. Diagnostic criteria for the classification of vocal cord dysfunction. *Chest* 2010; 138(5):1213-1223.

22. A. Nicotine transdermal patch.

SUBJECT: Tobacco use and dependence

Seven medications are currently approved by the Food and Drug Administration to treat tobacco dependency: bupropion SR, nicotine gum, nicotine inhaler, nicotine lozenge, nicotine nasal spray, nicotine patch, and varenicline. All of these medications have specific contraindications and precautions. Bupropion SR is a dopamine/norepinephrine reuptake inhibitor that has nicotinic cholinergic receptor antagonist properties. It is generally well tolerated with the most commonly reported side effects being insomnia and dry mouth. It is contraindicated in individuals with a history of seizures (answers B and C are incorrect), eating disorders, or taking another form of bupropion. Nicotine replacement therapy is highly effective in dependent smokers. The nicotine patch in particular has been shown to be safe for use in individuals with cardiovascular disease (answer D is incorrect). Nevertheless, it should still be used with caution in patients with recent myocardial infarction, unstable angina, or serious arrhythmias.

Although not listed as an option in this question, varenicline is a first line medication for treatment of tobacco dependency. It should be used with caution in patients with significant kidney disease (defined as a creatinine clearance less than 30 mL/min or receiving hemodialysis). Common side effects include insomnia and altered dream content. Since it has been on the market, there have been reports of change in mood, suicidal ideation, and even suicide in patients taking this medicine.

Fiore MC, Jaén CR, Baker TB, et al. Clinical practice guideline: Treating tobacco use and dependence: 2008 update. U.S. Department of Health and Human Services 2008 www.ahrq.gov.

23. B. Deep venous thrombosis.

SUBJECT: Deep venous thrombosis

It is difficult to make a clinical diagnosis of a deep venous thrombosis (DVT) based on presentation alone because the signs and symptoms are nonspecific. A broad differential diagnosis includes cellulitis, arthritis, muscle injury, lymphedema, chronic venous insufficiency, superficial thrombophlebitis, and popliteal cyst (Baker's cyst). The most common physical exam findings of an acute DVT include swelling, erythema, pain, and warmth. Calf pain with flexion of the knee and dorsiflexion of the ankle (Homan sign) and pain with calf compression against the tibia (Moses sign) are infrequently seen.

A clinical prediction model has been developed to assist in the evaluation of suspected DVT using the following variables:

- Active cancer treatment within the past 6 months (+1).
- Paralysis/paresis, or recent immobilization of the lower extremities (+1).
- Recently bedridden for 3 days or more, or major surgery within the past 12 weeks requiring general or regional anesthesia (+1).
- Localized tenderness along the distribution of the deep venous system (+1).
- Entire leg swelling (+1).
- Calf swelling at least 3 cm larger than that on the asymptomatic leg (measured 10 cm below the tibial tuberosity) (+1).
- Pitting edema confined to the symptomatic leg (+1).
- Collateral superficial veins (nonvaricose) (+1).
- Previously documented DVT (+1).
- Alternative diagnosis at least as likely as DVT (-2).

A score of 3 or greater indicates high probability, 1-2 moderate, and a score of 0 low probability for DVT. Individuals with a low probability have a prevalence of DVT less than 5%. When combined with a negative D-dimer, a DVT can be excluded without further workup. For patients with a probability other than low, or a positive D-dimer, additional workup is necessary.

Using the clinical prediction model, the individual in this question has a score of 3 (localized tenderness, pitting edema, and calf swelling 3 cm greater than the other leg). Therefore, a diagnosis of DVT should be pursued (answers A, C, and D are incorrect).

Wells PS, Owen C, Doucette S, et al. Does this patient have deep vein thrombosis? *JAMA* 2006;295:199-207.

24. B. Thoracotomy with right upper lobectomy and mediastinal lymph node dissection.

SUBJECT: Bronchial carcinoid tumor

Carcinoid tumors are derived from the neuroendocrine system. They are capable of secreting biologically active neuroamines and neuropeptides. While carcinoid tumors can arise from a number of organs, they are most commonly found in the digestive tract. Bronchial carcinoids make up 1% to 2% of all lung malignancies.

Proximal bronchial carcinoids usually present with cough and wheezing. Hemoptysis and postobstructive pneumonia may also occur. Peripheral lesions are more often asymptomatic and picked up incidentally. Bronchial carcinoid tumors are usually not associated with carcinoid syndrome, which consists of flushing, telangiectasia, diarrhea, and bronchoconstriction. Somatostatin receptor scintigraphy, serum chromogranin A, and 24-hour urine level of 5-hydoxyindoleacetic acid are not routinely performed unless there is a concern for metastatic disease. The individual in this question is asymptomatic and has normal laboratory data. Therefore, a search for metastatic disease is not indicated (answers A, C, and D are incorrect).

Historically carcinoid tumors were classified as typical or atypical. A typical carcinoid tumor consists of relatively bland cells with oval nuclei with scarce mitotic figures arranged in orderly nests (figure 24-C). In contrast an atypical carcinoid tumor has greater mitotic activity and the presence of necrosis.

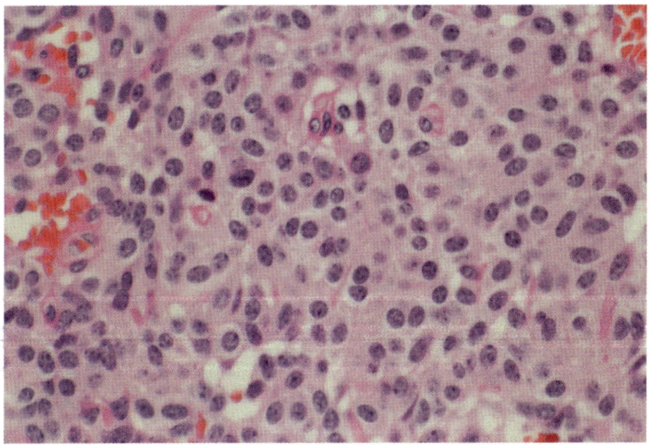

Figure 24-C

Detterback FC. Management of carcinoid tumors. *Ann Thorac Surg* 2010; 89:998-1005.

25. D. With appropriate treatment the syndrome will usually resolve within 24 hours.

SUBJECT: Tocolytic-induced pulmonary edema

Acute pulmonary edema can occur following the use of beta-adrenergic agents that are used to inhibit preterm labor. The condition develops in approximately 5% of pregnant women. Symptoms usually occur during or within 24 hours of treatment. Recognition of the syndrome is important since stopping the tocolytic agent is the primary treatment. Additional supportive care using supplemental oxygen and diuretics, if necessary, usually results in a rapid resolution of the condition (answer A is incorrect). Mechanical ventilation is generally not necessary (answer B is incorrect).

Potential risk factors for developing tocolytic-induced pulmonary edema include multiple pregnancies, diabetes, preeclampsia, blood transfusions, infections, simultaneous administration of magnesium sulfate, and use of glucocorticoids for more than 48 hours. Recommendations when using beta mimetic tocolytics include using the lowest possible perfusion rate, keeping the mother's heart rate at less than 100 beats/min, not using the agent for more than 48 hours, avoiding administration with other tocolytic drugs and magnesium sulfate, monitoring fluid balance closely, and avoiding use in high-risk individuals.

Pulmonary thromboembolic disease is the leading cause of unexpected maternal death (answer C is incorrect). Amniotic fluid embolism and peripartum cardiomyopathy are also significant causes of mortality.

Pereira A, Krieger BP. Pulmonary complications of pregnancy. *Clin Chest Med* 2004; 25:299-310.

26. C. Has a better prognosis than usual interstitial pneumonitis.

SUBJECT: Nonspecific interstitial pneumonitis

Nonspecific interstitial pneumonitis (NSIP) is one of the idiopathic interstitial pneumonias. The histologic features do not fit those seen with usual interstitial pneumonia, organizing pneumonia, desquamative interstitial pneumonia, lymphoid interstitial pneumonia, and acute interstitial pneumonitis. Cellular and fibrosing patterns of NSIP are recognized. The cellular pattern is characterized by mild/moderate interstitial chronic inflammation with Type II pneumocyte hyperplasia. Dense interstitial fibrosis is absent and organizing pneumonia is not prominent. The fibrosing pattern, which the patient in this question has, demonstrates features of dense fibrosis and lacks the temporal heterogeneity of usual interstitial pneumonia (figures 26-A and 26-B). Some cases show a mixture of both patterns. Conditions associated with NSIP include collagen vascular diseases, hypersensitivity pneumonitis, drug-induced pneumonitis, and infection. There is also an idiopathic form.

The clinical features of idiopathic NSIP are not well defined. Median age of onset is 40-50 years, and there is no gender predominance or association with cigarette smoking (answer B is incorrect). Dyspnea, cough, and fatigue are the usual presenting symptoms. Digital clubbing occurs less frequently than in patients with idiopathic pulmonary fibrosis. Pulmonary function testing typically shows a pattern of restriction with a reduced diffusion capacity (answer A is incorrect). Airflow obstruction is present in a minority of individuals. Chest computed tomography findings usually show the presence of ground glass attenuation, a feature that can be helpful in distinguishing it from usual interstitial pneumonitis. Honeycombing is usually minimal or absent (answer D is incorrect). The prognosis of NSIP is variable with some patients having a relatively stable course or even showing evidence of improvement. A minority of patients will progress and succumb to the disease.

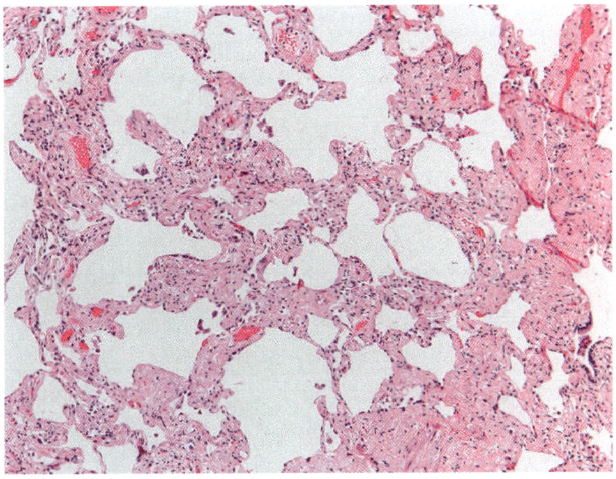

Figure 26-A

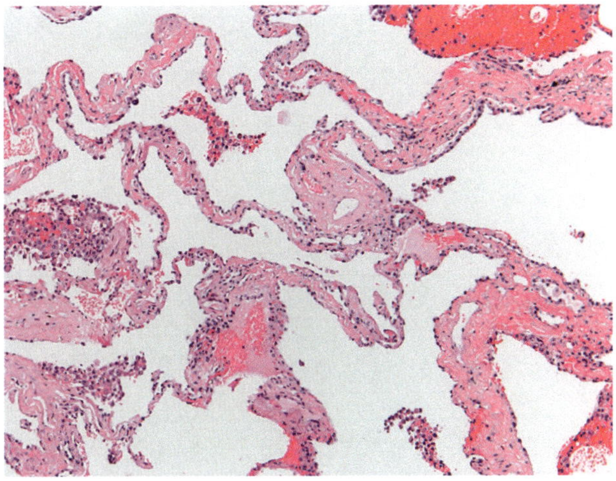

Figure 26-B

American Thoracic Society. American Thoracic Society/European Respiratory Society international multidisciplinary consensus classification of the idiopathic interstitial pneumonias. *Am J Respir Crit Care Med* 2002; 165:277-304.

27. C. Treatment with isoniazid, rifampin, pyrazinamide, and ethambutol.

SUBJECT: Tuberculous pleural effusion

The patient in this question has a tuberculous pleural effusion, a type of extrapulmonary tuberculosis (TB). The effusion can be either primary or due to reactivated disease. It is present in approximately 5% of patients infected with *Mycobacterium tuberculosis*. The pleural effusion is thought to be due to the rupture of a subpleural caseous focus from the lung into the pleural space resulting in a delayed hypersensitivity reaction. Although the effusion is the result of a hypersensitivity reaction, *M. tuberculosis* can usually be identified from culture of the fluid/pleural tissue. In contrast, a chronic TB empyema, which occurs less frequently than a TB pleural effusion, represents an active chronic infection of the pleural space. A TB pleural effusion usually manifests as an acute illness with the majority of patients being symptomatic for less than 1 month before seeking medical attention. Pleuritic chest pain and nonproductive cough are the main symptoms. The effusion is usually unilateral and small in size.

Thoracentesis typically shows clear to straw-colored fluid. It is usually not grossly bloody. The indices are compatible with an exudative process. Pleural fluid pH is usually 7.30 and 7.40. The glucose concentration is often > 60 mg/dL. During the early stage of illness, neutrophils may predominate, but there is a shift toward lymphocytosis the longer the effusion is present. Pleural fluid eosinophilia and > 5% mesothelial cells reduce the probability of the effusion being due to TB. Many of the effusions will spontaneously resolve within 1-4 months.

Diagnosis of a TB pleural effusion can be difficult. Direct examination of the pleural fluid detects acid-fast bacilli in a minority of cases. Culture increases the diagnostic yield, but it is still low (under 30%). Many lymphocyte pleural effusions have elevated adenosine deaminase (ADA) levels. An ADA level > 70 IU/L is suggestive of TB, while a level less than 40 IU/L nearly excludes the diagnosis. The highest diagnostic yield is obtained by thoracoscopy with parietal pleural biopsy and culture.

Patients with TB pleural effusion should be treated with a 4-drug regimen. Individuals who are positive for the human immunodeficiency virus are treated the same as those who are negative.

Because the patient is symptomatic and the indices on the pleural fluid are abnormal, observation is not appropriate (answer B is incorrect). Decortication is usually performed for conditions such as fibrothorax, empyema, and hemothorax (answer A is incorrect). The clinical presentation is not suggestive of venous thromboembolic disease, so proceeding with a ventilation-perfusion scan is not indicated (answer D is incorrect).

Gopi A, Madhavan SM, Sharma SK, et al. Diagnosis and treatment of tuberculous pleural effusion in 2006. *Chest* 2007; 131:880-889.

28. D. Perform behavior modification and dietary changes.

SUBJECT: Laryngopharyngeal reflux

Laryngopharyngeal reflux (LPR) refers to the back flow of stomach contents into the throat. In contrast, gastroesophageal reflux (GER) refers to the back flow of stomach content into the esophagus. These two conditions have different pathophysiological mechanisms, symptoms, and responses to treatment.

Patients with LPR typically do not complain of classic symptoms of esophagitis. Common symptoms of LPR include hoarseness, dysphagia, cough, throat clearing, and sore throat. Wheezing, postnasal drainage, excessive mucous in the throat, and a globus sensation are sometimes reported. It is believed that the primary abnormality in LPR is upper esophageal sphincter dysfunction. This is in contrast to GER where the primary defect is lower esophageal dysfunction.

The gold standard for the diagnosis of LPR is 24-hour dual probe pH monitoring. Barium esophagography and esophagoscopy are less sensitive. Oftentimes a clinical diagnosis is made based on symptoms and laryngeal findings. Optimal treatment for LPR is not yet defined. Patients with mild or intermittent symptoms are usually treated with dietary and lifestyle modifications. Patients are instructed to avoid caffeine, alcohol, peppermint, and acidic foods. More symptomatic patients require treatment with a histamine-2 antagonist or proton pump inhibitor. Pharmacologic therapy for LPR typically needs to be more aggressive and prolonged than for classic GER. The majority of patients with LPR usually require twice-daily proton pump inhibitor therapy for 6 months or longer.

Speech therapy and voice exercises are usually performed for treatment of vocal cord dysfunction (answer A is incorrect). The results of the bronchoprovocation test are more consistent with nonspecific bronchial hyperresponsiveness and not asthma. However, if a diagnosis of asthma was considered, the first line therapy would be an inhaled steroid and not a long-acting beta agonist (answer B is incorrect). Lisinopril can produce the side effect of cough, but not hoarseness or throat clearing. These symptoms suggest the patient's condition is not a medication side effect. Therefore, discontinuing lisinopril is not indicated (answer C is incorrect).

The chest radiographs in this question are normal.

Koufman JA, Aviv JE, Casiano RR, Shaw GY. Laryngopharyngeal reflux: Position statement of the committee on speech, voice, and swallowing disorders of the American Academy of Otolaryngology-Head and Neck Surgery. *Otolaryngol Head Neck Surg* 2002; 127:32-35.

29. A. Inspiratory muscle training.

SUBJECT: Pulmonary rehabilitation

There are several exercises that should be included in a pulmonary rehabilitation program. It is recommended that all programs include exercise training of the muscles of ambulation. Lower extremity exercise training at both low and high intensity is important with the latter producing greater physiologic benefits (answer B is incorrect). Unsupported endurance training of the upper extremities is also beneficial (answer C is incorrect). The addition of a strength training program has been shown to increase muscle mass and strength (answer D is incorrect). The available data do not support the routine use of inspiratory muscle training as an essential component of a rehabilitation program. There is also insufficient evidence to support the routine use of nutritional supplementation and anabolic steroids.

Ries AL, Bauldoff GS, Casaburi R, et al. Pulmonary rehabilitation: Joint ACCP/AACVPR evidence-based clinical practice guidelines. *Chest* 2007; 131:4S-42S.

30. C. The mortality rate is similar to other causes of acute lung injury.

SUBJECT: Transfusion-related acute lung injury

Transfusion-related acute lung injury (TRALI) occurs in temporal association with transfusion of blood products. To satisfy the criteria for a diagnosis, the patient must not have preexisting signs/symptoms of acute lung injury, have the onset of new lung injury within 6 hours after the end of a transfusion, and not have evidence of other conditions that could explain the acute lung injury. Virtually all blood components have been implicated in TRALI. This includes fresh frozen plasma, platelet concentrates, packed red blood cells, and whole blood. There are even reports of TRALI being precipitated by intravenous cryoprecipitate and immunoglobulins. There are different theories to explain TRALI. Leukocyte antibodies in the donor blood product may react to antigens on the recipient's granulocytes (answer A is a true statement). It has also been proposed that biologically active substances such as cytokines and lipids in the donor blood product may prime the recipient neutrophils (answer B is a true statement). The activated recipient neutrophils cause increased pulmonary capillary damage and leak leading to acute lung injury.

Clinical manifestations of TRALI include respiratory distress, hypoxemia, and occasionally hypotension. Mechanical ventilation is required in the majority of patients. With supportive care, the condition usually rapidly resolves within 3 days (answer D is a true statement). The mortality rate is approximately 5%, which is significantly lower than other causes of acute lung injury. If the recipient requires blood product transfusions in the future, it should be from a different donor. Blood products from other donors can be safely transfused.

Toy P, Popovsky MA, Abraham E, et al. Transfusion-related acute lung injury: Definition and review. *Crit Care Med* 2005; 33:721-726.

31. A. It is the result of a hypersensitivity pneumonitis.

SUBJECT: Nitrofurantoin-induced pulmonary toxicity

Pulmonary toxicity from nitrofurantoin can be either acute or chronic. The criteria for chronic nitrofurantoin-induced pulmonary toxicity include: one month or longer duration of respiratory symptoms, clinical and radiological evidence of lung disease, use of nitrofurantoin prior to the onset of symptoms, and exclusion of other causes of lung disease. The acute syndrome resembles a hypersensitivity pneumonitis with onset of fever, shortness of breath, and cough within 2 weeks of starting drug therapy. The chronic form is not due to a hypersensitivity mechanism. The syndrome may be the result of alveolar-epithelial injury from oxidative stress and immune-mediated responses.

Chronic nitrofurantoin-induced pulmonary toxicity usually presents with dyspnea, cough, and sometimes chest pain. Myalgias, fatigue, weight loss, and fever are typically not present. Inspiratory crackles may be present upon auscultation of the lungs. Digital clubbing is rare (answer B is a true statement). Laboratory abnormalities may include elevated liver enzymes and peripheral eosinophilia (answer C is a true statement). Pulmonary function testing usually shows evidence of restriction with a reduced diffusion capacity. Chest radiography typically shows diffuse, bilateral interstitial infiltrates. Pleural effusions are uncommon (answer D is a true statement). Surgical lung biopsy may show various patterns including nonspecific interstitial pneumonia, desquamative interstitial pneumonia, and organizing pneumonia.

Most patients with chronic nitrofurantoin-induced lung toxicity improve after drug withdrawal. However, residual radiographic abnormalities can persist. The use of glucocorticoid therapy as treatment remains controversial. There may be a role in the management of patients with severe symptoms although the dose and duration of therapy have not been defined.

Mendez JL, Nadrous HF, Hartman TE, et al. Chronic nitrofurantoin-induced lung disease. *Mayo Clin Proc* 2005; 80:1298-1302.

32. D. Lung biopsy will show features of diffuse alveolar damage.

SUBJECT: Acute interstitial pneumonitis

Acute interstitial pneumonitis (AIP) is one of the idiopathic interstitial pneumonias. It is defined by the onset of an acute lower respiratory tract illness within the prior 60 days, bilateral diffuse infiltrates on radiographic imaging, and the absence of any known inciting event. AIP appears to affect men and women equally with the mean age of onset of 54 years. Most individuals will present with a flu-like prodromal illness that escalates to fulminate respiratory failure usually requiring mechanical ventilation. The differential diagnosis includes acute eosinophilic pneumonia, acute cryptogenic organizing pneumonia, diffuse alveolar hemorrhage, drug-induced lung disease, acute hypersensitivity pneumonitis, infection, and exacerbation of usual interstitial pneumonia. Bronchoalveolar lavage typically shows a predominance of neutrophils and can be helpful in excluding conditions such as acute eosinophilic pneumonia, acute hypersensitivity pneumonitis, and diffuse alveolar hemorrhage syndromes. The characteristic finding on lung biopsy is the presence of diffuse alveolar damage (figures 32-A and 32-B). The injury is usually widespread and represents a mixture of inflammatory cells (predominantly mononuclear cells), proliferation of fibroblasts, Type II cell hyperplasia, interstitial edema, and hyaline membrane formation (the arrow in figure 32-A points to a hyaline membrane).

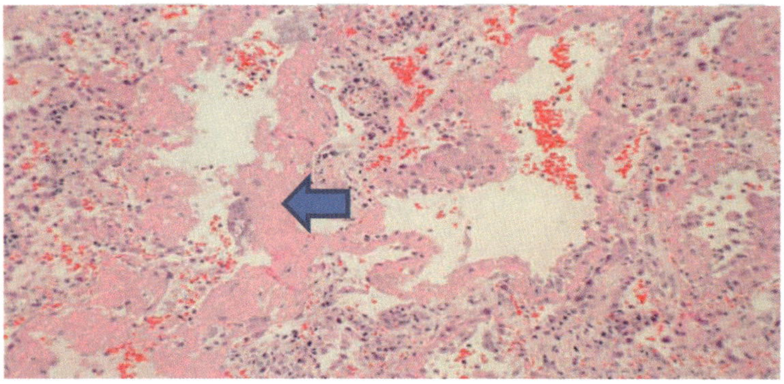

Figure 32-A

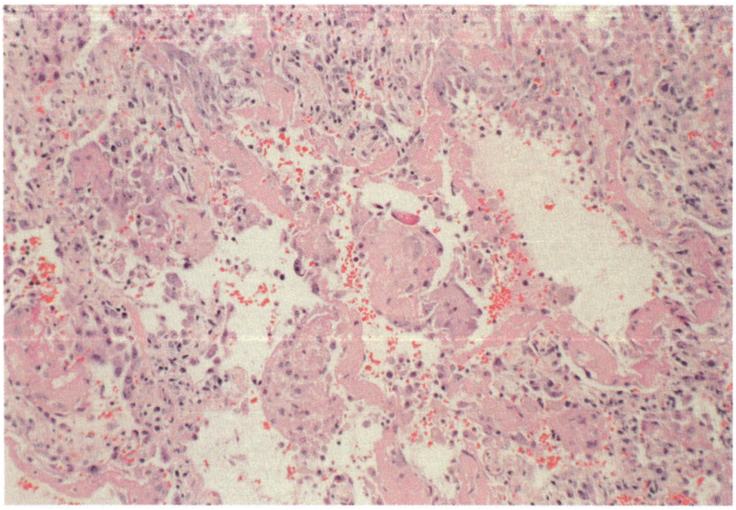

Figure 32-B

Treatment of AIP is mostly supportive. Glucocorticoids are usually administered at high doses although there is no proven survival benefit (answer A is incorrect). The overall mortality is approximately 70% (answer C is incorrect). Of the survivors, some will stabilize or show a recovery in lung function. Many, however, will experience relapse and have progression of disease (answer B is incorrect).

Vourlekis, JS. Acute interstitial pneumonia. *Clin Chest Med* 2004; 25:739-747.

33. B. Actinomycosis.

SUBJECT: Pulmonary actinomycosis

Actinomyces spp. are gram-positive, non-spore forming, predominately anaerobic bacteria that are commensals of the human oropharynx, gastrointestinal tract, and female genitalia. The typical symptoms of pulmonary actinomycosis are cough, sputum production, chest pain, dyspnea, and hemoptysis. Weight loss, malaise, night sweats, and fever can also be seen. The presentation can resemble other suppurative lung infections such as tuberculosis. An increased prevalence of the disease has been reported in individuals with underlying lung disease, alcoholism, and poor dentition.

Thoracic imaging studies are nonspecific, but often reveal a pneumonic lesion at the periphery of the lower lobes. This may reflect the possible role of aspiration in the pathogenesis of the disease. Diagnosis typically requires a lung biopsy for histological and microbiological confirmation. The histologic features show rounded basophilic masses capped by eosinophilic hyaline material. Foamy histiocytes and plasma cells are present. Giant cells are not present. The branching, gram-positive bacteria can be appreciated with tissue gram stain (see figure 33-C). The sulfur granule is the pathological hallmark of the disease. This lesion can be appreciated upon gross inspection and was originally thought to resemble elemental sulfur. Culturing the organism from sputum or bronchoalveolar fluid is inadequate for diagnosis as *Actinomyces* spp. can colonize the oropharynx. Penicillin is the drug of choice for treatment. Therapy may need to be continued for 6-12 months. Surgery should be considered if there are well-defined abscesses, empyema, or draining fistulas.

M. tuberculosis is a bacillus that stains positive with Gram's stain. *Nocardia* spp. are gram-positive, filamentous, branching rods. Both of these bacteria are acid-fast and therefore should be appreciated on specimens treated with the Kinyoun stain (answers C and D are incorrect). Malignant cells are not present on the biopsy (answer A is incorrect).

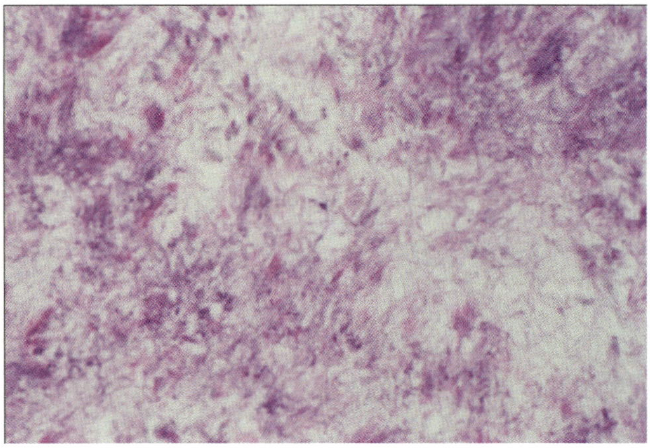

Figure 33-C

Mabeza GF, McFarlane J. Pulmonary actinomycosis. *Eur Respir J* 2003; 21:361-373.

34. D. Straw-colored fluid with less than 1,000/microL cells with a predominance of lymphocytes. Total protein concentration is 3.6 g/dL and the LDH is 150 U/L.

SUBJECT: Yellow nail syndrome

The classic triad of the yellow nail syndrome is lymphedema, pleural effusions, and yellow nails. The condition is thought to be the result of impaired lymphatic drainage. Approximately two-thirds of patients have pleuropulmonary symptoms. A history of chronic bronchitis, bronchiectasis, and pneumonia is often present. The pleural effusions are commonly bilateral and can range in size from small to massive. Thoracentesis should show straw-colored fluid. The total protein content is usually > 3 to 4 g/dL. The LDH is usually in the transudative range. Fluid pH and glucose should approximate serum levels. The fluid is commonly hypocellular with a predominance of lymphocytes.

There is no specific therapy for the yellow nail syndrome. Treatment is primarily supportive. Repeat therapeutic thoracentesis and even pleurodesis may be required for management of recurrent pleural effusions.

Answer A is the expected findings with a complicated parapneumonic effusion, answer B is seen with systemic lupus erythematosus, and answer C with a benign asbestos pleural effusion.

Hiller E, Rosenow EC, Olsen AM. Pulmonary manifestations of yellow nail syndrome. *Chest* 1972; 61:452-458.

35. A. Sarcoidosis.

<u>**SUBJECT**</u>: Lung transplantation

Several primary lung diseases have been reported to recur in the allograft. This includes sarcoidosis, bronchoalveolar cell carcinoma, desquamative interstitial pneumonitis, pulmonary alveolar proteinosis, giant cell interstitial pneumonitis, diffuse panbronchiolitis, talc granulomatosis, bronchiectasis secondary to aspiration, pulmonary Langerhans'- cell histiocytosis, and lymphangioleiomyomatosis.

Sarcoidosis is the most commonly reported disease to recur (answers B, C, and D are incorrect). The frequency has been reported to be as high as 35%. The reason for the high frequency is unknown, but it has been speculated that the formation of a sarcoid granuloma may share a common immune response with acute rejection. Recurrence of sarcoidosis has been reported as early as 2 weeks after transplantation. Most of the time the noncaseating granulomas are picked up incidentally when transbronchial biopsies are performed for surveillance of rejection. Chest computed tomography scanning in some cases of recurrence has documented the development of new interstitial densities and nodules.

Collins J, Hartman MJ, Warner TF, et al. Frequency and CT findings of recurrent disease after lung transplantation. *Radiology* 2001; 219:503-509.

36. A. Subglottic stenosis.

<u>**SUBJECT**</u>: Granulomatosis with polyangiitis

Granulomatosis with polyangiitis, formally known as Wegener's granulomatosis, is a systemic vasculitis with granulomatous inflammation most commonly involving the upper and lower respiratory tracts and kidneys. Other frequently involved body areas include joints, eyes, skin, nervous system, and heart.

Airway involvement is found in approximately 15% to 55% of patients. Several different tracheobronchial manifestations have been described. Subglottic stenosis is the most common. Bronchial stenosis does not occur frequently (answer B is incorrect). Areas of mucosal erythema, thickening, and ulceration are also frequently observed. Tracheal or bronchial polyps, tracheomalacia, and tracheobronchomalacia occur less commonly (answers C and D are incorrect).

Common presenting symptoms of lower respiratory tract airway involvement include hoarseness, stridor, wheezing, shortness of breath, and cough. Pulmonary function testing may be helpful in the evaluation of patients with these symptoms. The finding of a variable extrathoracic obstruction on the flow volume loop should raise suspicion of a subglottic lesion. The subglottic airway can easily be assessed with a bronchoscope. A number of nonmedical interventions can be used to manage subglottic stenosis. Therapies that have been used include balloon dilatation, laser ablation, tracheal stenting, and tracheostomy. There is no consensus regarding the optimal approach to treatment.

Polychronopoulos VS, Prakash UBS, Golbin JM, et al. Airway involvement in Wegener's granulomatosis. *Rheum Dis Clin N Am* 2007; 33:755-775.

37. D. Maximal expiratory pressure.

SUBJECT: Diaphragm paralysis

The patient in this question has unilateral diaphragm paralysis. The chest radiograph illustrates an elevated right diaphragm. The diaphragm is the main muscle of inspiration. Motor innervation is from the phrenic nerves that arise from the 3rd, 4th, and 5th cervical nerve roots. Unilateral paralysis is more common than bilateral paralysis. Most cases of unilateral paralysis are due to undetermined etiology. The differential diagnosis includes traumatic causes, neurologic disorders (such as multiple sclerosis, amyotrophic lateral sclerosis, poliomyelitis, and spinal cord transection), and myopathies (including systemic lupus erythematosus, inflammatory myopathies, and amyloidosis). Many patients with unilateral diaphragm dysfunction are asymptomatic. Some will complain of dyspnea with exertion. If both diaphragms are involved, severe dyspnea and orthopnea are typically present. These individuals are also at risk for a sleep-related hypoventilation/hypoxic syndrome.

Spirometry usually demonstrates a vital capacity that is about 75% of predicted with unilateral paralysis, and less than 50% of predicted with bilateral paralysis (answer A is incorrect). The supine vital capacity is characteristically less than the upright value (answer B is incorrect). Because the diaphragm is an inspiratory muscle, the maximal inspiratory pressure will be reduced (answer C is incorrect). The maximal expiratory pressure will be normal.

Qureshi A. Diaphragm paralysis. *Semin Respir Crit Care Med* 2009; 30:315-320.

38. A. The individual is most likely a non-smoker.

SUBJECT: Hypersensitivity pneumonitis

Hypersensitivity pneumonitis (HP) results from an abnormal inflammation of the lung parenchyma in response to inhalation of a specific antigen that the individual has been previously sensitized to.

The major antigens responsible for causing HP include fungi, bacteria, bird proteins, and an assortment of different chemicals. A recreational history obtained in this case led to a diagnosis of "hot tub lung." This form of HP develops when an individual is exposed to the microorganisms from the *Mycobacterium* genus that can reside in hot tubs.

The clinical presentation of HP is traditionally classified as acute, subacute, and chronic. The acute form is thought to be most common and is characterized by the onset of symptoms within several hours following antigen exposure. Symptoms can include dyspnea, cough, chest tightness, and extrapulmonary symptoms of fever and chills. The diagnosis can be challenging as the syndrome can mimic viral and bacterial infections. Significant predicators of HP include exposure to a known offending antigen, recurrent episodes, onset of symptoms within 4 to 8 hours after exposure, weight loss, inspiratory crackles on physical examination, and the presence of positive precipitating antibodies. Smoking is not a risk factor for HP, unlike with other parenchymal lung diseases such as desquamative interstitial pneumonitis, pulmonary Langerhans' -cell histiocytosis, and respiratory bronchiolitis-associated interstitial lung disease.

The role of measuring serum precipitins in HP remains controversial. HP cannot be diagnosed solely on the basis of positive antibodies (answer D is incorrect). Many asymptomatic individuals will have a positive test result. Likewise, the absence of specific antibodies does not exclude a diagnosis of HP. The presence of specific antibodies should be used only as supportive evidence for a diagnosis. Analysis of bronchoalveolar lavage fluid is helpful in the diagnosis of HP. Marked lymphocytosis should be present. Lymphocyte subset analysis should reveal a CD4/CD8 ratio < 1 (answer C is incorrect). There are no findings on lung biopsy that are unique to HP. The presence of poorly formed noncaseating granulomas has been described in HP. Patterns of nonspecific interstitial pneumonitis, organizing pneumonia, and usual interstitial pneumonitis are more likely to be seen in subacute or chronic cases.

The primary treatment is antigen avoidance. Systemic glucocorticoids may hasten recovery from an acute episode in highly symptomatic patients. While there is also interest in the use of chronic glucocorticoids to suppress inflammation in subacute and chronic cases of HP, it is unclear if the long-term course of the disease is altered. Furthermore, side effects of treatment may further complicate management.

Exhaled nitric oxide has been mostly studied in the management of asthma. It has been looked at in other conditions such as bronchiectasis and chronic obstructive pulmonary disease, but not as a way to monitor disease course in HP (answer B is incorrect).

Lacasse Y, Girard M, Cormier Y. Recent advances in hypersensitivity pneumonitis. *Chest* 2012; 142:208-217.

39. D. Bronchial artery embolization.

SUBJECT: Aspergilloma

An aspergilloma is a fungal ball that is contained within a lung cavity. Individuals with Stage IV sarcoidosis are at risk for this complication. Asymptomatic individuals may be closely observed. However, the onset of hemoptysis can be an ominous sign. It is usually due to local vascular invasion of the cavity wall by the fungus. The optimal treatment for hemoptysis is uncertain. Endobronchial catheter placement with installation of Amphotericin B or a sclerosing agent has not been shown to be highly effective (answer B is incorrect). While surgery is considered curative, patients with preexisting lung disease are oftentimes not surgical candidates. The patient in this question is a poor surgical candidate because of his pulmonary function test and cardiopulmonary exercise test results (answer A is incorrect). Bronchial artery embolization may successfully stop acute bleeding. Even if this is successful, there is a risk of re-bleeding in the future. Percutaneous installation of antifungal antibiotics into the cavity has been performed with limited success. Systemic antifungal therapy is generally not beneficial because of the lack of blood supply, but could be considered in patients who have a component of semi-invasive disease (answer C is incorrect).

Limper AH, Knox KS, Sarosi GA, et al. An official American Thoracic Society statement: Treatment of fungal infections in adult pulmonary and critical care patients. *Am J Respir Crit Care Med* 2011; 183:96–128.

40. C. Dysphonia.

SUBJECT: Side effects of inhaled glucocorticoids

The most common local side effect of inhaled glucocorticoids is dysphonia (answers A, B, and D are incorrect). The etiology is most likely steroid myopathy affecting the vocal cord muscles. It is reversible with discontinuation of therapy.

Other local side effects of inhaled glucocorticoids include perioral dermatitis, oropharyngeal candidiasis, tongue hypertrophy, cough, and sensation of thirst. Because some of the medicine is swallowed, there is also a risk for systemic complications. Such problems can include risk for osteoporosis, adrenocortical suppression, skin bruising, posterior subcapsular cataracts, and glaucoma. The risk is greatest when high-potency glucocorticoids are used for prolonged periods. Slit lamp eye examination and bone densitometry should be considered in at-risk individuals.

Roland NJ, Bhalla RK, Earis J. The local side effects of inhaled corticosteroids. *Chest* 2004; 126:213–219.

41. D. Ischemic heart disease.

SUBJECT: Chronic obstructive pulmonary disease and cardiovascular mortality

Coronary artery disease and COPD frequently coexist because of the shared common risk factor of tobacco use. However, it also turns out that reduced lung function and chronic bronchitis, regardless of smoking history, are independent predicators of the occurrence of ischemic heart disease. The rate of hospitalization for cardiovascular disease complications is higher than that for COPD itself. COPD has also been linked to hypertension, ventricular arrhythmias, supraventricular arrhythmias, and stroke. Cardiovascular disease-related morbidity and mortality are nearly twice as high in patients with COPD as in the general population. The presence of cardiovascular disease predicts all-cause mortality in patients with COPD. Ischemic heart disease causes more deaths than do respiratory complications of COPD, bronchogenic carcinoma (answer A is incorrect), bacterial pneumonia (answer B is incorrect), and pulmonary embolism (answer C is incorrect).

Selective beta-blockers (atenolol, metoprolol) appear to be safe and have a low risk of serious side effects when used in individuals with COPD. Nonselective beta-blockers have a higher likelihood of precipitating bronchospasm.

Huiart L, Ernst P, Suissa S. Cardiovascular morbidity and mortality in COPD. *Chest* 2005; 128:2640-2646.

42. B. Pleural effusion.

SUBJECT: Pulmonary embolism and chest radiograph findings

The majority of patients with an acute pulmonary embolism (PE) will have an abnormality identified on chest radiographs. Pleural effusion is common, occurring in nearly 50% of patients with documented PE. Although not listed as an option in this question, nonspecific atelectasis may be more common.

The majority of pleural effusions due to a PE are small and usually of no clinical significance. Most will spontaneously resolve within 1 to 3 weeks. Thoracentesis is not warranted unless the effusion is moderate to large in size or there is uncertainty about the diagnosis. When performed, the pleural fluid can be of variable characteristics. The majority will have exudative features. The presence of a hemorrhagic effusion is not a contraindication to anticoagulation. Less than 25% of patients will have a transudative effusion.

Less common radiographic abnormalities include the Westermark sign, which is a focal area of avascularity (answer A is incorrect), the Hampton hump, which is a pleural-based, wedge-shaped density (answer D is incorrect), and the Fleischner sign, which refers to prominence of the central pulmonary artery (answer C is incorrect).

Yap E, Anderson G, Donald J, et al. Pleural effusion in patients with pulmonary embolism. *Respirology* 2008; 13:832-836.

43. A. Nausea, vomiting, anorexia, constipation, lethargy, and dehydration.

SUBJECT: Squamous cell carcinoma of the lung

A paraneoplastic syndrome results from the metabolic activity remote from the primary tumor. Syndromes can be classified as neurologic, skeletal, renal, hematologic, cutaneous, and endocrinologic. Squamous cell carcinoma of the lung can cause hypercalcemia, which the patient in this question has. The biopsy shows features of keratization and intercellular bridges. It may arise from bone metastases or secretion of a parathyroid hormone-related protein. The latter causes accelerated bone reabsorption and renal calcium reabsorption. Symptoms include nausea, vomiting, constipation, anorexia, lethargy, polydipsia, polyuria, and dehydration.

Digital clubbing and hypertrophic osteoarthropathy most commonly occur with adenocarcinoma of the lung (answer A is incorrect). Carcinoid tumors can produce a syndrome that causes coughing, wheezing, cutaneous flushing, and diarrhea (answer C is incorrect). Cancer associated retinopathy is most commonly due to small cell carcinoma and presents with painless bilateral vision loss, ring scotomas, night blindness, and photosensitivity (answer D is incorrect).

Heinemann S, Zabel P, Hauber, H-P. Paraneoplastic syndromes in lung cancer. *Cancer Ther* 2008; 6:687-698.

44. D. Isoniazid, rifabutine, pyrazinamide, and ethambutol daily for 8 weeks followed by isoniazid and rifabutine twice weekly for 18 weeks.

SUBJECT: Acquired immunodeficiency deficiency syndrome and pulmonary tuberculosis

In general, treatment for tuberculosis in adults infected with HIV is similar to HIV-uninfected adults. There are some important exceptions. Rifampin has interactions with many antiretroviral agents that can adversely affect HIV treatment. A rifampin-based TB regimen is usually used when the patient is receiving the nonnucleoside reverse transcriptase inhibitor efavirenz along with two nucleoside analogs. Administration with protease inhibitors, which the patient in this question is taking, is not recommended. Therefore, rifabutine must be substituted as the rifamycin of choice. There is also a risk of resistance with rifamycin use, and therefore any continuation phase regimens that administer rifamycins twice weekly or less are contraindicated. The regimens in answers A, B, and C are acceptable to use.

Some patients with HIV-related tuberculosis will experience an immune reconstitution syndrome while being treated with antituberculosis agents. The syndrome is characterized as a temporary worsening of symptoms and radiographic findings. The optimal treatment for this has not been defined. Supportive treatment using nonsteroidal anti-inflammatory agents may be beneficial in some patients.

Centers for Disease Control and Prevention. Treatment for tuberculosis, American Thoracic Society, CDC, and Infectious Diseases Society of America. *MMWR* 2003; 52:1-79.

45. C. Admission to the intensive care unit.

SUBJECT: Asthma and pregnancy

During pregnancy, asthma control can be highly variable. A general rule is that it will improve in one-third of patients, worsen in one-third of patients, and remain the same in one-third of patients. Maternal asthma can increase the risk of placenta previa, preeclampsia, and maternal hospital stay. Adverse effects on the infant can include low birth weight, preterm delivery, and lengthened infant hospital stay. Asthma that is well controlled reduces these risks.

Inhaled glucocorticoids are the foundation of asthma treatment during pregnancy. The Food and Drug Administration has labeled inhaled budesonide a class B medication (no evidence of risk in studies). Other inhaled glucocorticoids are designated class C (risk cannot be ruled out) but are generally considered safe to be used during pregnancy. Inhaled glucocorticoids used at appropriate doses do not appear to impair intrauterine growth of the fetus. During acute exacerbations, systemic glucocorticoids should be used.

A number of physiologic changes occur with pregnancy that will affect respiratory function. There is normally an increase in minute ventilation that results in a respiratory alkalosis. A normal $PaCO_2$ during pregnancy varies between 28 mm Hg and 32 mm Hg. Arterial pH is usually between 7.40 and 7.47. Eucapnia in a pregnant woman should be interpreted as possible impending respiratory failure, which is why the patient in this question should be admitted to the intensive care unit (answers A, B, and D are incorrect).

Namazy JA, Schatz M. Pregnancy and asthma: recent developments. *Curr Opin Pulm Med* 2005; 11:56-60.

46. C. Secondary pulmonary hypertension is usually mild and of no clinical significance.

SUBJECT: Pulmonary Langerhans' -cell histiocytosis

Langerhans' cells are differentiated cells of monocyte-macrophage lineage. These cells can infiltrate different organs. The term pulmonary Langerhans' -cell histiocytosis refers to lung involvement that can occur in isolation or in addition to other organ involvement. A minority of individuals will have extrapulmonary organ involvement (answer D is incorrect). For example, 5% to 15% of patients with pulmonary Langerhans' -cell histiocytosis will have hypothalamic involvement giving rise to diabetes insipidus, cutaneous involvement causing a rash, or adenopathy due to lymph node involvement. The Langerhans' cell has some unique histopathologic features. The first is the presence of Birbeck granules, which are pentilaminar intracytoplasmic inclusions. Langerhans' cells also express CD1 antigen and S100 protein.

The incidence and prevalence of pulmonary Langerhans' -cell histiocytosis has not been well defined. It is thought to be a rare disorder and probably affects men and women equally. The only consistent risk factor is cigarette smoking. While many patients are found to have this condition incidentally, common presenting symptoms include nonproductive cough, dyspnea, fever, night sweats, and anorexia. Symptoms may also be dictated by other organ involvement. Spontaneous pneumothorax is frequently a presenting symptom (answer A is incorrect).

High-resolution computed tomography usually shows nodular and cystic changes with a predilection for the middle and upper lobes bilaterally. The cysts are usually thin-walled. The presence of classic features on high-resolution computed tomography scanning is highly suggestive of Langerhans' -cell histiocytosis. Bronchoscopy with bronchoalveolar lavage is expected to show CD1a positive cells. Greater than 5% CD1a positive cells is considered diagnostic (answer B is incorrect). Levels less than this are indeterminate. Performing a transbronchial biopsy is usually low yield because of the patchy nature of the disease. The highest diagnostic yield is obtained with a surgical biopsy. The proliferation of Langerhans' cells leads to formation of nodules. The nodules have a stellate appearance and are comprised of other cell populations including eosinophils, lymphocytes, plasma cells, fibroblasts, and macrophages (figures 46-C and 46-D). Because most of these patients also smoke, illnesses such as respiratory bronchiolitis-interstitial lung disease or desquamative interstitial pneumonitis may also be evident on the biopsy.

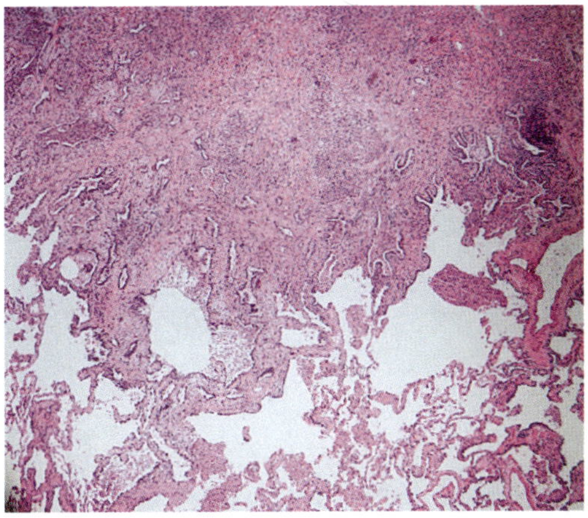

Figure 46-C

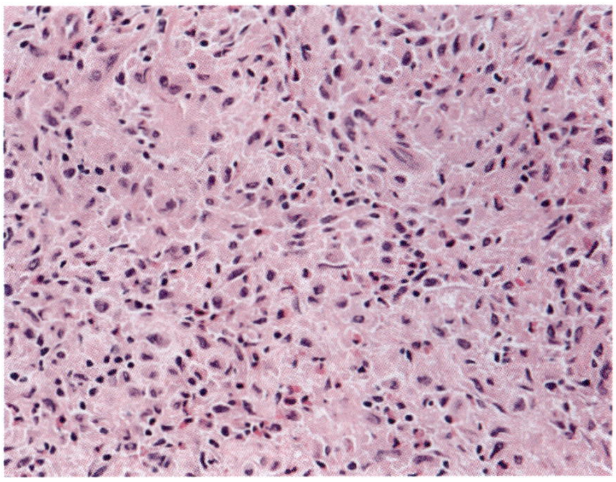

Figure 46-D

The primary treatment is smoking cessation. There are limited data supporting the efficacy for routine use of glucocorticoids. Nevertheless, a trial is usually given to patients with progressive disease. Lung transplantation has been used in patients with end-stage disease. Several findings are associated with a poor prognosis including advanced age, multi-organ involvement, honeycombing, and pulmonary hypertension. In patients with advanced disease the degree of pulmonary hypertension is almost always severe and associated with increased mortality. The association between pulmonary Langerhans' -cell histiocytosis and malignant neoplasms is unclear. There may be an increased incidence of lymphoma and bronchogenic carcinoma.

Vassallo R, Ryu JH, Colby TV, et al. Pulmonary Langerhans' -cell histiocytosis. *N Engl J Med* 2000; 342:1969-1978.

47. C. Endovascular stent placement.

<u>**SUBJECT**</u>: Fibrosing mediastinitis

The patient in this question has fibrosing mediastinitis leading to the superior vena cava syndrome. The symptoms and physical examination findings, including a positive Pemberton's sign (sensation of head congestion, dizziness, or fullness with extension of the arms above the head) and Kussmaul's sign (neck vein distention with inspiration) are the result of impeded venous outflow. Fibrosing mediastinitis is due to chronic inflammation and a subsequent fibrotic reaction. The extensive fibrosis can encase mediastinal lymph nodes and invade into the adjacent mediastinal structures. It is most commonly due to prior infection from *Histoplasmosis capsulatum*. It is not the result of ongoing active infection but rather thought to be due to leakage of fungal antigen from infected lymph nodes into the mediastinal space leading to a chronic hypersensitivity reaction.

A number of complications can occur from fibrosing mediastinitis. Bronchial airway involvement can lead to problems such as postobstructive pneumonia, broncholithiasis, and hemoptysis. Superior vena cava obstruction is common. Obstruction of the pulmonary arteries can result in secondary pulmonary hypertension and cor pulmonale. Esophageal involvement can lead to dysphagia.

Computed tomography scanning of the chest is useful in the evaluation of patients with fibrosing mediastinitis. There is usually a characteristic pattern of a fibrous mass with calcification. The extent of involvement of great vessels and mediastinal organs can be assessed. Biopsy is usually not indicated and may carry with it a high risk of bleeding complications. It should be performed only in cases where the diagnosis is unclear. The prognosis is highly variable. Many individuals will have a chronic stable course while others will experience significant morbidity and early mortality. There is no specific treatment that has been shown to be highly effective. There is no established role for antifungal therapy or systemic glucocorticoids (answers A and B are incorrect). Surgery can sometimes be performed to relieve airway obstruction. There is no established role for radiation therapy (answer D is incorrect). Endovascular stenting of an artery or vein can be performed to relieve vascular obstruction. Endobronchial stenting should be considered if there is significant airway involvement.

Wheat LJ, Conces D, Allen SD, et al. Pulmonary histoplasmosis syndromes: Recognition, diagnosis, and management. *Semin Respir Crit Care Med* 2004; 25:129-144.

48. A. During the first few minutes of exercise there is an initial bronchoconstriction.

SUBJECT: Exercise-induced bronchospasm

The patient in this question has exercise-induced bronchospasm (EIB). The cardiac findings are consistent with a benign apical systolic murmur that is common in healthy children. The majority of asthmatics have some degree of EIB. During the first 1-3 minutes of exercise, the airways initially dilate (answer B is incorrect). The initial bronchodilation is followed by a period of bronchoconstriction that starts minutes into the exercise period. It generally peaks within 10-15 minutes and then will gradually wane and usually resolve within 60 minutes (answer C is incorrect). Repeated exertion will cause less bronchoconstriction (answer D is incorrect). The increase in minute ventilation that occurs with exercise results in heat and water loss from the airways. The subsequent cooling and dryness of the airways causes bronchospasm. EIB is less when the inspired air is humidified and closer to body temperature.

An accurate diagnosis of EIB should include objective documentation of bronchial hyperresponsiveness. This might include use of a bronchoprovocation test with methacholine or a laboratory-based exercise challenge using either a treadmill or cycle ergometer. A 10% fall in the FEV_1 following an exercise challenge is considered positive. Recommended treatment for EIB includes the use of an inhaled short-acting beta agonist prior to exercise. A warm-up period before heavy exertion may also reduce the degree of bronchospasm. Cromolyn or nedocromil taken before exercise are alternatives to short-acting beta agonists but not as effective. Leukotriene receptor antagonists can also attenuate EIB. Frequent or severe episodes may warrant a step-up in therapy with consideration of scheduled inhaled glucocorticoids.

Parsons JP, Mastronarde JG. Exercise-induced asthma. *Curr Opin Pulm Med* 2009; 15:25–28.

49. B. It is an autosomal recessive disease.

<u>SUBJECT</u>: Primary ciliary dyskinesia

Primary ciliary dyskinesia (PCD) is an autosomal recessive disease. The principle defect is a congenital impairment in the cilia. A number of different defects have been described. Clinical manifestations typically include chronic rhinosinusitis, recurrent otitis media, nasal polyposis, bronchiectasis, and infertility. Most males are infertile. While some women can successfully conceive a child and carry it to term, the majority cannot (answer D is incorrect). Individuals with PCD have a normal lifespan (answer C is incorrect). Some individuals with PCD have the triad of situs inversus, chronic sinusitis, and bronchiectasis, referred to as Kartagener's syndrome. The chest radiograph in this question demonstrates situs inversus totalis.

High-resolution computed tomography scanning of the chest sometimes reveals saccular or cylindrical bronchiectasis (answer A is incorrect). Traction bronchiectasis occurs in the setting of diffuse parenchymal lung diseases such as usual interstitial pneumonitis.

Bush A, Cole P, Hariri M, et al. Primary ciliary dyskinesia: diagnosis and standards of care. *Eur Respir J* 1998; 12:982–988.

50. A. Nifedipine.

<u>SUBJECT</u>: High altitude pulmonary edema

Ascent to a high altitude is not without risk. High altitude illness is a phrase that encompasses a number of syndromes such as acute mountain sickness, high altitude cerebral edema, and high altitude pulmonary edema. High altitude pulmonary edema refers to the noncardiogenic accumulation of fluid within the alveoli. Host factors, rate of ascent, and the degree of altitude all are risk factors. Pulmonary edema usually occurs at elevations greater than 2,500 m but can also occur below this. The primary prevention is gradual ascent. With respect to preventive pharmacologic therapy, nifedipine is the drug of choice. It should be prescribed a day prior to ascent and possibly continued until a descent below 2,500 m.

Acetazolamide is the agent of choice for the prevention of acute mountain sickness (answer B is incorrect). Dexamethasone is an alternative agent. Neither has been well studied for prevention of high altitude pulmonary edema. Phosphodisterase 5 inhibitors and beta agonists also await further investigation before their use can be recommended (answers C and D are incorrect).

Hackett PH, Roach RC. High altitude illness. *N Engl J Med* 2001; 345:107-114.

51. D. Hepatic failure.

<u>SUBJECT</u>: Bleomycin-induced pulmonary toxicity

Bleomycin is commonly used in the treatment of lymphomas, germ cell tumors, and head and neck malignancies. Several distinct pulmonary toxicity syndromes have been reported including hypersensitivity pneumonitis, organizing pneumonia, acute chest pain syndrome with drug infusion, and interstitial pneumonitis. There is a risk of progressing to chronic fibrosis with the interstitial pneumonitis form of toxicity. Patients with bleomycin-induced interstitial pneumonitis usually present with dry cough, dyspnea, and sometimes fever. Several risk factors have been identified including cumulative drug dose (answer A is incorrect), age greater than 70, renal impairment (answer C is incorrect), smoking (answer B is incorrect), and administration of supplemental oxygen. Hepatic dysfunction does not increase the risk for toxicity.

The diagnosis of bleomycin-induced interstitial pneumonitis is usually one of exclusion. If there is a concern for pulmonary infection, bronchoscopy with bronchoalveolar lavage should be performed. Treatment consists primarily of drug discontinuation and supportive care. Individuals with organizing pneumonia or a hypersensitivity reaction to bleomycin will respond favorably to glucocorticoids.

Whether or not glucocorticoids change the course of interstitial pneumonitis is uncertain. The mortality of patients with interstitial pneumonitis is approximately 3%.

Sleijfer S. Bleomycin-induced pneumonias. *Chest* 2001; 120:617-624.

52. D. Relapses are common but not associated with increased mortality or functional morbidity.

SUBJECT: Cryptogenic organizing pneumonia

Organizing pneumonia is a pattern of lung injury that can be seen in a number of conditions including bacterial, viral, parasitic, and fungal infections, drug reaction, secondary to lung transplantation or bone marrow grafting, gastroesophageal reflux, and connective tissue diseases. If no cause is identified, the condition is referred to as cryptogenic organizing pneumonia (COP). The classic histologic features of organizing pneumonia include proliferation of granulation tissue within the small airways, alveolar ducts, and alveoli. Features of vasculitis, granulomatous inflammation, and necrosis are absent (figure 52-C. The arrow points to an area of granulation tissue).

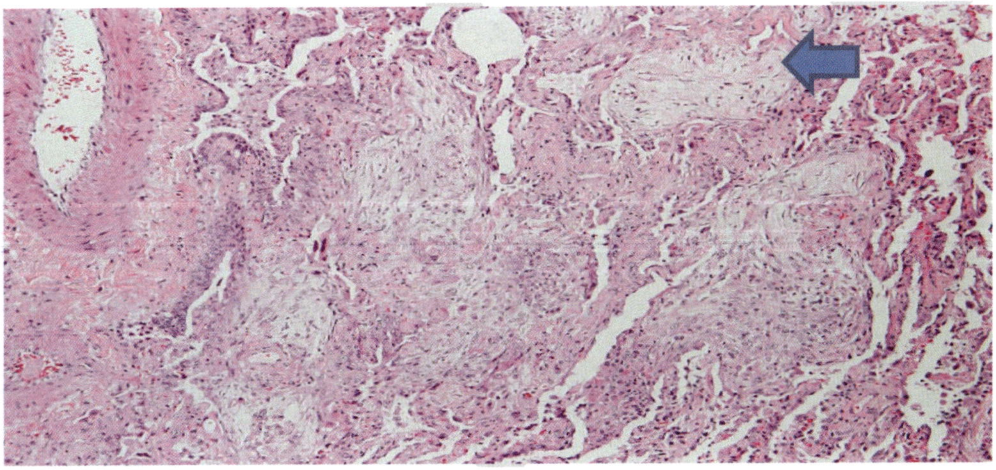

Figure 52-C

COP occurs in males and females equally with a mean age of onset between 50 and 60 years. The disorder is not related to smoking. Patients usually present with a mild flu-like illness followed by progressive dyspnea, anorexia, and weight loss. Hemoptysis is uncommon (answer A is incorrect). Chest pain, night sweats, and arthralgia are also typically not seen. Physical examination may be normal or show sparse crackles. Imaging studies may show different patterns, such as multiple alveolar opacities with a patchy peripheral bilateral distribution. The condition may also present as a solitary opacity or infiltrative processes. Honeycombing is absent. Bronchoalveolar lavage is helpful in excluding other diagnoses. The differential cell count is nonspecific but may include increased alveolar macrophages, lymphocytes, and neutrophils. Abundant eosinophils should not be present and if so would point to an alternative diagnosis. A confident diagnosis requires lung biopsy. Transbronchial biopsies are usually insufficient to characterize the intraalveolar buds (answer B is incorrect). Video-assisted thorascopic surgery with biopsies is usually required to make a confident diagnosis.

Glucocorticoid treatment typically results in rapid clinical improvement with resolution of symptoms and chest radiograph abnormalities (answer C is incorrect). Relapses are common upon tapering or stopping glucocorticoids, and therefore long-term treatment is often indicated. Relapses are not associated with increased mortality or functional morbidity.

Cordier, JF. Cryptogenic organising pneumonia. *Eur Respir J* 2006; 28:422-446.

53. A. The patient has contact with birds.

SUBJECT: Psittacosis

Psittacosis (also referred to as ornithosis) is due to infection by *Chlamydophila psittaci.* Birds are the main reservoir for the organism. Virtually all common domestic as well as wild birds can carry *C. psittaci.* Transmission to humans primarily occurs following inhalation of the organism shed in bird secretions or excretions. Although much more rare, infection of humans from mammals such as sheep and cats can also occur. The onset of the disease is characterized by high fever, headache, myalgias, and cough. Arthralgias, mental status changes, and gastrointestinal disturbances may also be present. A variety of skin manifestations such as erythema nodosum and a diffuse, pale, macular rash (Horder's spots) can also occur. Uncommon manifestations of psittacosis include endocarditis, pericarditis, meningitis, and spontaneous abortion. A variety of laboratory abnormalities have been described including leukocytosis, elevated liver function tests, and hyponatremia.

The treatment of choice for psittacosis is one of the tetracyclines. Macrolides are a second line therapy. Penicillin is not effective (answer B is incorrect).

Seasonal influenza has a peak incidence in the Northern Hemisphere during the winter months (answer C is incorrect). Hospital-acquired cases of Legionnaires' disease have been linked to *Legionella* spp. in the water supply (answer D is incorrect).

Grayston JT, Thom DH. The chlamydial pneumonias. *Curr Clin Top Infect Dis* 1991; 11:1-18.

54. B. The pleural fluid indices are likely to have exudative characteristics.

SUBJECT: Systemic lupus erythematosus-related pleural effusion

Systemic lupus erythematosus (SLE) is an autoimmune disorder that can affect virtually every organ system. The most common pulmonary manifestation is pleurisy with or without pleural effusions. When present, the effusions are usually bilateral and small. A moderate to large unilateral effusion is not characteristic of SLE-related pleural disease (answer C is incorrect). The pleural effusion indices typically have exudative characteristics. Antinuclear antibody, anti-DNA antibodies, and LE cells may be present in the pleural fluid. LE cells are thought to be specific for a lupus pleural effusion. The LE cell is a mature polymorphic nuclear leukocyte that has phagocytized nuclear material. It is very difficult to identify and is not present in all pleural effusions. An ANA > 1:40 and a pleural fluid/serum ANA > 1 are suggestive of SLE but not diagnostic (answer A is incorrect). Treatment options are dictated by the severity of symptoms. Asymptomatic effusions can oftentimes be observed. For more severe disease, glucocorticoids or disease modifying agents should be considered. Invasive procedures including pleurodesis are generally not required (answer D is incorrect).

Other pulmonary manifestations of SLE include chronic interstitial pneumonitis, acute lupus pneumonitis, diffuse alveolar hemorrhage, pulmonary hypertension, thromboembolism, diaphragm dysfunction, and infection in individuals receiving immunosuppressive therapy.

Keane MP, Lynch JP. Pleuropulmonary manifestations of systemic lupus erythematosus. *Thorax* 2000; 55:159-166.

55. C. Continue prednisone, tacrolimus, and azathioprine but all at reduced dosages.

SUBJECT: Posttransplant lymphoproliferative disorder

Posttransplant lymphoproliferative disorders (PTLD) can occur following solid organ transplantation. The major risk factor is thought to be Epstein-Barr virus (EBV) negative serology prior to transplantation and subsequent EBV seroconversion after transplantation. Intense immunosuppression is also a risk factor. The reported incidence following lung transplantation varies widely between 2% and 20%.

PTLD represents a spectrum of disorders ranging from benign polyclonal lymphoid proliferation to malignant lymphoma. The patient in this question has the former condition. Most cases will present within the first year after transplant. Radiographic patterns at the time of presentation range from a solitary pulmonary nodule to multiple nodules with mediastinal adenopathy. Extrapulmonary metastases may also occur.

The primary treatment is to reduce the immunosuppression (answer B is incorrect). The use of the CD20 monoclonal antibody rituximab has shown promise. The use of chemotherapy or radiation is not been well defined (answer A is incorrect). There may be a role for these treatments in Hodgkin lymphoma-like PTLD. It is unknown if the incidence of PTLD can be significantly decreased with the administration of prophylactic antivirals. Agents such as ganciclovir are not currently being used as primary treatment of PTLD (answer D is incorrect).

Reams BD, McAdams P, Howell DN, et al. Posttransplant lymphoproliferative disorder. *Chest* 2003; 124:1242-1249.

56. C. Plasmapheresis, prednisone, and cyclophosphamide.

SUBJECT: Antiglomerular basement membrane antibody syndrome

Antiglomerular basement membrane antibody syndrome (Goodpasture's syndrome) is the result of antibodies directed against the NC1 domain of the alpha 3 chain of the basement collagen type 4. The syndrome is characterized by diffuse alveolar hemorrhage and glomerulonephritis. The former can present with hemoptysis, anemia, diffuse pulmonary infiltrates, and hypoxemic respiratory failure. In 10% of the cases, there is no renal involvement. Males are more commonly affected than females. The majority of cases occur between the ages of 20 and 30. The condition is more common in smokers. The histopathologic changes in the lungs are that of bland hemorrhage, although capillaritis has been described.

Treatment consists of concurrent plasmapheresis, glucocorticoids, and cyclophosphamide (answers A and B are incorrect). Plasmapheresis removes circulating antibodies while the glucocorticoids and cyclophosphamide prevent new antibody generation. The duration of treatment is determined by clinical response and measuring serial levels of circulating antiglomerular basement antibodies. Antibody levels will usually be undetectable after a few weeks of treatment. Longer treatment is needed if the levels remain elevated. Enuretic patients may require dialysis and even kidney transplantation. The patient in this question is not enuretic and has no other indications for dialysis (answer D is incorrect). Although the prognosis has improved with treatment, death due to diffuse alveolar hemorrhage can still occur.

Lara AR, Schwarz MI. Diffuse alveolar hemorrhage. *Chest* 2010; 137:1164-1171.

57. B. Early institution of NIPPV may result in an improvement in the quality of life and a survival benefit.

SUBJECT: Amyotrophic lateral sclerosis

Amyotrophic lateral sclerosis (ALS) is a progressive neurodegenerative disease affecting motor neurons in the motor cortex, brainstem, and spinal cord. There is a spectrum of manifestations with the primary clinical symptoms determined by the specific motor neurons involved. Most deaths from ALS are due to respiratory failure.

The FVC is the most commonly used respiratory measurement to assess pulmonary function in individuals with ALS. It is a strong predictor of survival. The supine FVC is a better predictor of diaphragm weakness than the upright FVC. A decrease to 50% of predicted or less is associated with significant respiratory symptoms. The FVC, however, does not correlate well with the presence of nocturnal hypoventilation. Nocturnal oximetry, maximal inspiratory pressure, and the sniff nasal pressure may be more sensitive at detecting the onset of respiratory insufficiency, hypercapnia, and nocturnal hypoxemia.

Noninvasive positive pressure ventilation (NIPPV) should be considered in ALS patients with an FVC less than 50% of predicted, abnormal nocturnal oximetry, maximal inspiratory pressure less than -60 cm, sniff nasal pressure less than 40 cm, and in those experiencing orthopnea. There are data showing that NIPPV improves survival in selected patients with ALS, particularly in those individuals without bulbar involvement, such as the patient in this example. The benefit to those with poor bulbar function is not well established (answer D is incorrect). NIPPV has also been shown to improve quality of life and slow the rate of FVC decline (answer A is incorrect).

Relative contraindications to long-term use of NIPPV include the inability to protect the airway, excessive secretions, poorly motivated patient/family, inability to cooperate with treatment, and the need for continuous or nearly continuous ventilatory assistance. The patient in this question does not have a contraindication to using NIPPV (answer C is incorrect).

Miller RG, Jackson CE, Kasarskis EJ, et al. Practice parameter update: The care of the patient with amyotrophic lateral sclerosis: Drug, nutrition, and respiratory therapies (an evidence-based review). *Neurology* 2009; 73:1218-1226.

58. D. Areas of normal lung alternating with areas of dense collagen, scattered foci of fibroblastic proliferation, and cystic fibrotic air spaces. Hyaline membranes are absent.

SUBJECT: Hermansky-Pudlak syndrome

Hermansky-Pudlak syndrome is a rare autosomal recessive disease. Several different subtypes have been described. The syndrome is characterized by oculocutaneous albinism and hemorrhagic defects due to platelet dysfunction. Certain disease manifestations are thought to be the end result of the accumulation of a ceroid-like material in various tissues. Hermansky-Pudlak syndrome is also associated with pulmonary fibrosis. The average age of onset of lung disease is in the 4th decade. Symptoms usually occur insidiously. The course can be progressive and lead to death. Lung biopsy will show histologic features of usual interstitial pneumonitis, which includes areas of normal lung alternating with areas of dense collagen, scattered foci of fibroblastic proliferation, and cystic fibrotic air spaces. Hyaline membranes should be absent. Macrophages filled with a ceroid-like material may be present.

Answer B is characteristic of diffuse alveolar damage, answer C has the hallmarks of diffuse alveolar hemorrhage, and answer A has the histologic features of lymphangioleiomyomatosis.

White DA, Walker Smith GJ, Copper JAD, et al. Hermansky-Pudlak syndrome and interstitial lung disease: Report of a case with lavage findings. *Am Rev Respir Dis* 1984; 130:138-141.

59. A. Coronavirus.

SUBJECT: Severe acute respiratory syndrome

The human coronaviruses are a common cause of an acute respiratory illness known simply as the common cold. The offending organism is spread through respiratory secretions. In 2003, a new coronavirus was responsible for an illness characterized by fever, chills, malaise, headache, and myalgias, followed by the acute respiratory distress syndrome. Diagnostic studies showed lymphopenia, thrombocytopenia, elevated lactate dehydrogenase, and elevated transaminases. The illness became known as severe acute respiratory syndrome. It was associated with significant mortality.

The Sin Nombre virus, a hantavirus, is responsible for an acute cardiopulmonary syndrome. Following a 2-3-week incubation period, the affected individual will have a prodromal illness characterized by fever, chills, myalgia, and gastrointestinal disturbances manifesting as nausea, vomiting, and diarrhea. This is followed by a cardiopulmonary phase with pulmonary edema causing respiratory failure and hemodynamic collapse. Laboratory data shows leukocytosis with a marked left shift and circulating immunoblasts. Thrombocytopenia and hemoconcentration are frequently present (answer B is incorrect).

Influenza virus infection is characterized by an abrupt onset of fever, chills, sore throat, headache, myalgia, nasal congestion, and anorexia. Laboratory abnormalities include elevated transaminases, anemia, and elevated creatinine kinase. The course is frequently complicated by a secondary bacterial infection by organisms such as *Streptococcus pneumoniae* and *Staphylococcus aureus* (answer C is incorrect).

Adenovirus usually causes a syndrome characterized by fever, rhinitis, pharyngitis, keratoconjunctivitis, tracheitis, bronchitis, and pneumonia (answer D is incorrect).

Peiris JSM, Phil D, Yuen KY, et al. The severe acute respiratory syndrome. *N Eng J Med* 2003; 349:2431-41.

60. A. Schedule ciclesonide 80 mcg two inhalations twice daily.

SUBJECT: Mild persistent asthma

The patient in this question has mild persistent asthma. For individuals > 12 years of age, mild persistent asthma is defined as symptoms occurring greater than 2 days/week but not daily, nighttime awakenings 3-4 times/month, use of a short-acting beta agonist for symptom control greater than 2 times/week but not daily and not more than 1 time on any day. Symptoms cause a minor limitation to normal activity. The FEV_1 should be greater than 80% of predicted, and the FEV_1/FVC ratio should be normal.

The preferred treatment for mild persistent asthma is use of a low dose of inhaled glucocorticoids. Alternative therapies include cromolyn, a leukotriene receptor antagonist, nedocromil, or theophylline. Increasing the use of the patient's short-acting beta agonist would not be appropriate (answer B is incorrect).

A number of conditions can worsen asthma control including exercise, viral infections, inhalant allergens, environmental irritants, changes in weather, menstrual cycle, stress, strong emotional expressions, certain medications, and comorbid conditions such as sinusitis, rhinitis, and gastroesophageal reflux. Although the individual in this question has a history of gastroesophageal reflux, the condition is well controlled with lifestyle modification, and instituting medical treatment is therefore not indicated as the next most appropriate therapy for the patient in this question (answers C and D are incorrect).

National Institutes of Health. Guidelines for the diagnosis and management of asthma. *National Asthma Education and Prevention Program Expert Panel Report 3* 2007. www.nhibi.gov/guidelines/asthma.

61. D. Periodic spirometry after initiation of therapy should not be used to monitor disease status in stable patients.

SUBJECT: Chronic obstructive pulmonary disease diagnosis and management

History and physical examination are poor predictors for the presence and severity of airflow obstruction. Spirometry is a simple, cost-effective method to identify airflow obstruction. A diagnosis of COPD is confirmed when a symptomatic patient has evidence of airflow obstruction defined as a postbronchodilator FEV_1/FVC of < 0.70.

The evidence does not support the use of spirometry as a screening tool for airflow obstruction in at-risk individuals who are asymptomatic (answer B is incorrect). Patients who appear to benefit the most from inhaled bronchodilators (anticholinergic or long-acting beta agonists) are those with symptoms and an FEV_1 less than 60% of predicted (answer A is incorrect). The specific choice of therapy may depend on patient preference, cost issues, and risk of adverse effects. There is no evidence to support the routine use of intermittent spirometry after the initiation of therapy to monitor disease status. Sharing spirometry findings with a patient has not been shown to independently improve the likelihood of smoking cessation or continued abstinence (answer C is incorrect).

Qaseem A, Wilt TJ, Weinberger SE, et al. Diagnosis and management of stable chronic obstructive pulmonary disease: A clinical practice guideline update from the American College of Physicians, American College of Chest Physicians, American Thoracic Society, and European Respiratory Society. *Ann Intern Med* 2011; 155:179-191.

62. C. Electrocardiogram.

SUBJECT: D-dimer

The patient in this question has viral pericarditis. A pericardial friction rub can be appreciated at end expiration. Early electrocardiogram findings will show ST elevation in all leads except reciprocal depression in aVr, along with PR segment depression, flattening of T-waves, and diminished voltage of the QRS complex.

An elevated D-dimer can be seen in the following situations: venous thromboembolic disease, disseminated intravascular coagulopathy, eclampsia, arterial thromboembolic disease, sepsis, congestive heart failure, surgery, trauma, cancer, renal disease, and pregnancy. The finding of an elevated D-dimer should not always be an automatic prompt to pursue a diagnosis of pulmonary embolism (answers A, B, and D are incorrect).

Stein PD, Hull RD, Patel KC, et al. D-dimer for the exclusion of acute venous thrombosis and pulmonary embolism, A systemic review. *Ann Intern Med* 2004; 140:589.

63. B. Repetitive nerve stimulation of an involved muscle will show a decrease in the compound muscle action potential.

SUBJECT: Small cell lung cancer

The patient in this question has a small cell lung cancer causing the Lambert-Eaton syndrome. The biopsy shows small, round, blue cells with scant cytoplasm, nuclear molding, and necrosis (figures 63-B and 63-C). This paraneoplastic syndrome has also been described with myeloproliferative conditions. It is a result of antibodies directed against the voltage-gated calcium channel at the presynaptic nerve terminal. This causes a decrease in the amount of acetylcholine release.

Presenting symptoms of Lambert-Eaton syndrome commonly include weakness of the proximal muscles, diminished deep tendon reflexes, abnormal gait, and ptosis. Autonomic manifestations including dry mouth, erectile dysfunction in males, and constipation are common.

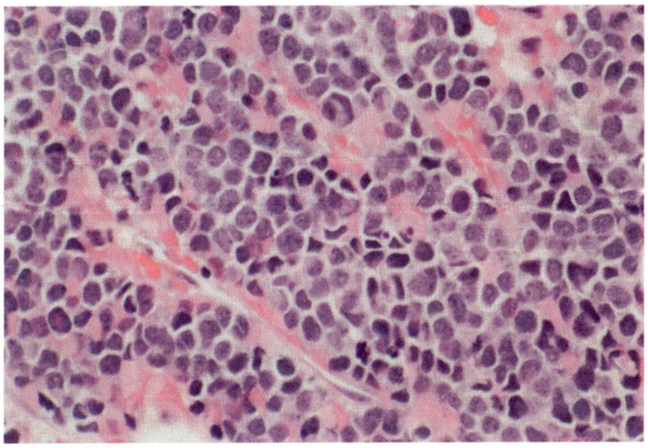

Figure 63-B

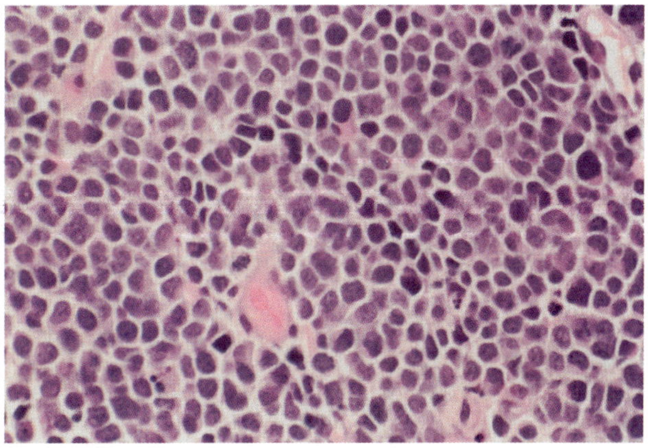

Figure 63-C

Lambert-Eaton syndrome must be differentiated from myasthenia gravis. The latter is a result of antibodies against the postsynaptic membrane acetylcholine receptor. Ocular, bulbar, and respiratory muscle groups are frequently affected. Lambert-Eaton syndrome can be diagnosed by demonstrating a high antibody titer against P/Q-type voltage-gated calcium channel (answer C is a true statement). Neurophysiologic patterns are also useful in the diagnosis. Following maximal isometric contraction, muscle strength and deep tendon reflexes will temporarily improve (answer D is a true statement). Electrical stimulation of an involved muscle group will show an increase in the compound muscle action potential (answer A is a true statement). In contrast, a decrease in the potential is seen in individuals with myasthenia gravis.

Titulaer MJ, Wirtz PW, Kuks JB, et al. The Lambert-Eaton myasthenic syndrome 1998-2008: A clinical picture in 97 patients. *J Neuroimmunol*; 2008:153-158.

64. A. Cigarette smoking has been established as a causative agent.

SUBJECT: Acute eosinophilic pneumonia

Acute eosinophilic pneumonia (AEP) tends to occur more often in men than in women with an average age of onset between 19 and 37 years. Approximately two-thirds of individuals are current smokers. A relationship between the onset of cigarette smoking and the development of AEP has been shown. In fact, several patients have undergone a smoking provocation test with the recurrence of AEP symptoms within hours of smoking. AEP has also been described following the exposure to tear gas, gasoline, firewood smoke, and cocaine. Asthma is not recognized as a risk factor (answer B is incorrect).

The diagnosis of AEP requires that the following criteria be satisfied: acute onset of a febrile illness that is present less than 1 month in duration, bilateral diffuse infiltrates on chest radiographs, hypoxic respiratory failure ($P_aO_2 < 60$ mm Hg, or arterial oxygen saturation < 90% on room air), bronchoalveolar lavage showing > 25% eosinophils or eosinophilic pneumonia on tissue biopsy, and the absence of other known causes of pulmonary eosinophilia. Blood eosinophilia, if at all present, is typically mild at the time of presentation. Chest radiographs usually show bilateral ground glass opacities.

AEP uniformly responds to the administration of glucocorticoids. There is no consensus as to the optimal dose and duration of treatment. Spontaneous relapse of AEP has not been documented (answer C is incorrect).

There is nothing in this case history to suggest a helminthic infection. When such an infection is suspected, a diagnosis can usually be made with serologic testing. Analyzing stool can be low yield as the larvae are secreted intermittently. Stool analysis in this example will be normal (answer D is incorrect).

Janz DR, O'Neal HR, Ely EW. Acute eosinophilic pneumonia: A case report and review of the literature. *Crit Care Med* 2009; 37:1470-1474.

65. D. Observation.

SUBJECT: Coccidiomycosis

The fungi *Coccidioides immitis* and *Coccidioides posadasii* are responsible for coccidiomycosis. These soil-dwelling fungi are localized to regions of the Western Hemisphere. The San Joaquin Valley of California and parts of Arizona are endemic regions within the United States. The majority of cases occur by inhalation. Nearly two-thirds of infections are asymptomatic. Those who are symptomatic have an illness similar to community-acquired bacterial pneumonia. Less than 1% of the cases result in disseminated disease. Risk factors for dissemination include male gender, race (blacks), diabetes mellitus, ethnicity (Filipinos and Native Americans), congestive heart failure, chronic renal failure, pregnancy, chronic obstructive pulmonary disease, and human immunodeficiency virus infection. Chest radiographs initially show a patchy pneumonitis and associated ipsilateral hilar adenopathy. Discreet nodules mimicking malignancy may sometimes be present. Lesions can undergo central necrosis to form a thin-walled cavity. It may take 1 to several months after infection for cavity formation.

Immunocompetent patients do not require any specific treatment for primary pulmonary coccidiomycosis (answers A and B are incorrect). Therapy should be considered if symptoms persist for more than 6 weeks or for severe acute disease. When treatment is indicated, fluconazole or itraconazole are the agents of choice for pulmonary disease. Amphotericin B products are reserved for severe disease. In contrast, all immunosuppressed patients should be considered for treatment. Isoniazid, rifampin, ethambutol, and pyrazinamide are used in the treatment of tuberculosis, not coccidiomycosis (answer C is incorrect).

Limper AH, Knox KS, Sarosi GA, et al. An official American Thoracic Society statement: Treatment of fungal infections in adult pulmonary and critical care patients. *Am J Respir Crit Care Med* 2011; 183:96-128.

66. C. Reduces airborne dust mite and cockroach particles.

SUBJECT: Asthma control

Indoor air cleaning devices such as HEPA and electrostatic precipitating filters can reduce airborne allergens from dogs, cats, mold spores, and particulate tobacco smoke (answers A, B, and D are true statements). They are not really effective for reducing dust mite and cockroach particles as these substances do not remain airborne. Most studies do not show any effect on symptom control or lung function with use of these filters.

Measures to reduce dust mites include encasing pillows and mattresses in a special dust mite-proof cover and washing the pillow, sheets, and blankets each week in hot water. Use of dehumidifiers or central air conditions to reduce indoor humidity to below 60%, removing carpets from the bedroom, and keeping stuffed toys out of the bed are other simple measures that can be performed.

To reduce exposure to cockroaches, all food and garbage should be kept in closed containers. Cockroach baits/traps are also effective.

National Institutes of Health. Guidelines for the diagnosis and management of asthma. *National Asthma Education and Prevention Program Expert Panel Report 3* 2007. www.nhlbi.gov/guidelines/asthma.

67. D. An oral glucocorticoid once daily.

SUBJECT: Cystic fibrosis treatment

Airway clearance methods, mucolytic agents, bronchodilators, and anti-inflammatory therapies all have a role in the treatment of individuals with cystic fibrosis (CF). A number of different airway clearance methods can be used such as chest physiotherapy, positive expiratory pressure devices, autogenic drainage, and high-frequency chest wall oscillation systems (answer A is a correct treatment). There are no data showing that one method is superior to the others. Treatment should be individualized.

Recombinant human dornase alpha decreases the viscosity of sputum. Use of this agent has been shown to result in an improvement in pulmonary function, decrease in respiratory tract infections, fewer hospital days, and need for fewer days receiving parenteral antibiotics (answer B is a correct treatment). There are no data supporting the routine use of alternative mucolytic agents such as N-acetylcystine or hypertonic saline.

Bronchodilators are commonly used in the treatment of CF as the majority of patients have bronchial hyperreactivity. A fast-onset beta-2-adrenergic receptor agonist can improve symptoms and possibly pulmonary function (answer C is a correct treatment). Anticholinergic bronchodilators, theophylline, and long-acting beta agonists may be beneficial in selected patients. Inhaled short-acting bronchodilators are usually administrated prior to use of an airway clearance device or exercise to assist with removal of secretions.

There is also interest in the use of anti-inflammatory therapies in patients with CF. The use of high-dose ibuprofen therapy (up to 1,600 mg orally twice daily) has been shown to slow the progression of pulmonary disease in patients with an FEV_1 > 60% of predicted. This is most pronounced in children between the ages of 5 and 12 years. There are not data showing a benefit in individuals with more severe disease. The use of ibuprofen is limited because of potential gastrointestinal and renal toxicities. The use of systemic glucocorticoids is discouraged because of the potential risks such as cataracts, glucose intolerance, and osteoporosis. Even an every-other-day regimen is not advised. The only possible exception to this would be in individuals whose course is complicated by allergic bronchopulmonary aspergillosis. The routine use of inhaled glucocorticoids is not recommended.

Yankaskas JR, Marshall BC, Sufian B, et al. Cystic fibrosis adult care. *Chest* 2004; 125:1S-39S.

68. B. Begin antibiotic therapy with intravenous vancomycin.

SUBJECT: Sickle cell disease and the acute chest pain syndrome

Sickle cell disease is a common autosomal recessive disorder. The substitution of valine for glutamic acid at position 6 in the beta globin chain of hemoglobin A results in hemoglobin S. The inheritance of 2 defective beta globin genes is the cause of sickle cell disease. The polymerization of hemoglobin S leads to hemolysis and vasoocclusive episodes. The acute chest syndrome, which the patient in this question is experiencing, is a type of lung injury that occurs during a vasoocclusive crisis.

The acute chest syndrome is characterized by fever, chest pain, tachypnea, cough, and new pulmonary infiltrates. It is associated with significant morbidity and premature death. The main causes of the acute chest pain syndrome are pulmonary infection, in situ thrombosis of the pulmonary vasculature, and embolization of bone marrow fat. Respiratory infections are most commonly due to pathogens such as *Chlamydia pneumoniae*, *Mycoplasma pneumoniae*, and respiratory viruses. Infection with *Staphylococcus aureus* and *Streptococcus pneumoniae* are less common. When antibiotics are administered, they should cover the more common bacterial pathogens; therefore, the administration of vancomycin would not be appropriate.

Use of incentive spirometry has been shown to prevent atelectasis and alveolar hypoxia during an acute chest pain crisis (answer A is a true statement). Transfusion of red blood cells to a hemoglobin level > 11 g/dL has been associated with complications of viscosity (answer C is a true statement). Correction of hypoxia is important. Supplemental oxygen should be administered to achieve an oxygen saturation that is > 92% (answer D is a true statement).

Another common pulmonary complication of sickle cell disease is pulmonary hypertension. There is an association between the development of pulmonary hypertension and the severity of hemolytic anemia. Pulmonary hypertension has also been described in other chronic hereditary and acquired hemolytic anemias.

Galdwin MT, Vichinsky E. Pulmonary complications of sickle cell disease. *N Engl J Med* 2008; 359:2254-2265.

69. B. Discontinue amiodarone.

SUBJECT: Amiodarone-induced pulmonary toxicity

The incidence of amiodarone-induced pulmonary toxicity is estimated to be between 5% and 13%. Risk factors for toxicity include a daily dose > 400 mg for longer than 2 months, increased patient age, underlying lung disease, thoracic/nonthoracic surgery, and pulmonary angiography.

A number of different pulmonary manifestations have been described, including organizing pneumonia, acute respiratory distress syndrome (ARDS), interstitial pneumonitis, pleural effusions, hypersensitivity pneumonitis, and nodules/masses. A form of chronic pneumonitis, which can lead to fibrosis, has also been described This condition usually presents with insidious onset of shortness of breath, dry cough, weight loss, and occasionally fever. Pulmonary function testing will demonstrate a restrictive ventilator defect with a reduced diffusion capacity. Imaging studies commonly show diffuse, patchy infiltrates bilaterally. Physical examination may show inspiratory crackles but is otherwise unremarkable. Lung biopsy findings are nonspecific but characteristically show interstitial inflammation, fibrosis, Type II pneumocytes, and the presence of foamy alveolar macrophages (figures 69-B and 69-C. The arrow points to a group of foamy macrophages).

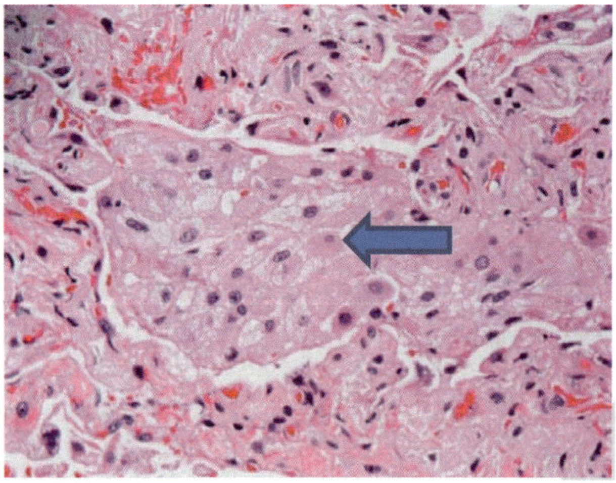

Figure 69-B

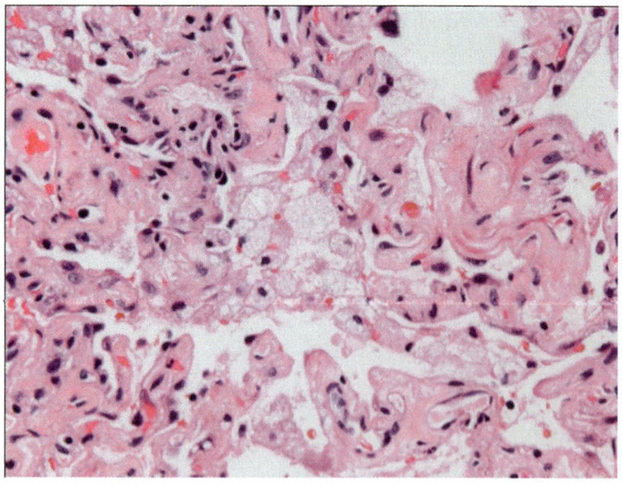

Figure 69-C

The primary treatment of amiodarone-induced pulmonary toxicity is drug withdrawal. Most cases have a good prognosis with the overall mortality less than 10%. Individuals who develop ARDS and require mechanical ventilation, however, have a mortality rate greater than 50%. There is no consensus about the use of glucocorticoids for treatment, although a trial is typically given for patients who are acutely ill (answer D is incorrect).

There is no evidence this patient has tuberculosis (answer A is incorrect). There is no indication for lobectomy to be performed (answer C is incorrect).

Pourafkari L, Ghaffari MR, Yaghoubi, A, et al. Amiodarone-induced lung toxicity. *J Cardiovasc Thorac Res* 2010; 2:1-4.

70. C. Nitrogen dioxide.

SUBJECT: Bronchiolitis

Bronchioles are small airways (< 2 mm) that do not contain cartilage. Bronchiolitis is a general term that implies inflammation of the bronchioles. There is significant confusion surrounding this term. This is made worse by the different classification systems used for bronchiolar diseases. For example, a clinical classification system recognizes disorders due to inhalation injury, drug toxicity, infection, and idiopathic. A histopathological classification system recognizes constrictive bronchiolitis, proliferative bronchiolitis, follicular bronchiolitis, and diffuse panbronchiolitis.

Constrictive bronchiolitis, also known as obliterative bronchiolitis and bronchiolitis obliterans, is characterized by a pattern of peribronchiolar fibrosis resulting in complete narrowing of the bronchiolar lumen. The lesions are typically patchy and may be missed due to sampling error. Transbronchial biopsy is therefore usually not diagnostic. Surgical lung biopsy is required to make a confident diagnosis. Disorders associated with constrictive bronchiolitis include infection (mostly due to respiratory viruses), connective tissue disease, inhalation injury, allograft recipients, drugs, and other disorders such as inflammatory bowel diseases. The patient in this question was a farmer with exposure to nitrogen dioxide from a grain bin.

Patients with constrictive bronchiolitis usually present with cough and dyspnea. Inspiratory crackles can sometimes be appreciated upon auscultation. Pulmonary function tests show airway obstruction, air trapping, and a normal or decreased diffusion capacity. High-resolution computed tomography of the chest at complete end expiration should be performed in the evaluation of bronchiolar disorders. The usually finding is mosaic areas of decreased attenuation and vascularity with regions of air trapping.

Bronchioles may have dilated lumens or thickened walls. In most cases, constrictive bronchiolitis tends to be progressive. Although glucocorticoids are often used for treatment, the response is variable.

Exposure to thermophilic actinomycetes and bird protein antigen can lead to hypersensitivity pneumonitis. The histopathologic abnormalities may include poorly formed granulomas associated with a mononuclear infiltration (answers B and D are incorrect). Isocyanates are associated with occupational asthma (answer A is incorrect).

Ryu JH, Myers JL, Swensen SJ. Bronchiolar disorders. *Am J Respir Crit Care Med* 2003; 168:1277–1292.

71. C. Admission to the hospital general medical ward and start oral levofloxacin.

SUBJECT: Community-acquired pneumonia

Severity-of-illness scores can be used to assist with decision making for disposition of patients with community-acquired pneumonia. The CURB-65 (confusion, urea higher than 20 mg/dL, respiratory rate ≥ 30 breaths/min, low blood pressure defined as systolic < 90 mm Hg or diastolic ≤ 60 mm Hg, and age ≥ 65 years) is one such severity-of-illness score. Each patient characteristic is assigned 1 point value. The 30-day mortality for 0 to 1 point is 1.5%, 2 points 9.2%, and 3-5 points 22%. A CURB-65 score of 0–1 can be treated as an outpatient, whereas those with a score of 2 should be admitted to the hospital ward. Patients with a score of ≥3 should go to the intensive care unit. The patient in this question has a score of 2 based on age and blood urea nitrogen level and should be admitted to the general medical ward (answers A, B, and D are incorrect). For inpatients not requiring intensive care unit treatment, a respiratory quinolone or a beta lactam plus a macrolide would be adequate antibiotic therapy.

Mandell LA, Wunderink RG, Anzueto A, et al. Infectious Diseases Society of America/American Thoracic Society consensus guidelines on the management of community-acquired pneumonia in adults. *Clin Infect Dis* 2007; 44:S27–72.

72. A. Take additional occupational history.

SUBJECT: Benign asbestos-related pleural effusion

A benign asbestos-related pleural effusion (BAPE) is one of the more common nonmalignant conditions related to asbestos exposure. Asbestos minerals can be found in a number of products such as brake lining, pipes, pillars, tiles, shipyards, and insulation. The patient in this question served in the navy for 5 years. Prior to 1970, navy ships were heavily insulated with asbestos. Many sailors were exposed while serving their country. A BAPE oftentimes occurs earlier (within 10 years) following exposure to asbestos, in contrast to the other asbestos-related diseases that have a longer latency. The pathogenesis of BAPE is not well understood, but may be the result of asbestos fibers migrating from the lung into the parietal pleura and instigating a pleuritis. Patients are usually asymptomatic, although fever and pleuritic chest pain may be present.

A BAPE is usually unilateral and small to moderate in size. The fluid is characteristically an exudate and frequently hemorrhagic. Pleural fluid eosinophilia can be present. Most effusions will persist for several months and then spontaneously resolve. Some effusions will reoccur. The diagnosis is one of exclusion. Patients suspected of having a BAPE should be followed to confirm the benign nature of the condition.

In this example the occupational history lead to a confident presumptive diagnosis of BAPE. Therefore, pursuing other diagnoses with additional invasive testing is not warranted (answers C and D are incorrect). While tuberculosis can cause an exudative pleural effusion, fluid eosinophilia is uncommon. Microbiologic or histologic confirmation of infection should be sought before initiating treatment (answer B is incorrect).

American Thoracic Society. Diagnosis and initial management of nonmalignant diseases related to asbestos. *Am J Respir Crit Care Med* 2004; 170:691-715.

73. C. Administration of colchicine postoperatively may have prevented this illness.

SUBJECT: Postpericardiotomy syndrome

The postcardiac injury syndromes include postmyocardial infarction syndrome (Dressler's syndrome), postpericardiotomy syndrome, and posttraumatic pericarditis. Damage to the cells of the pericardium or myocardium results in a release of antigens that stimulates an immune reaction. Immune complexes subsequently deposit in the pericardium, pleura, and lungs.

The diagnosis of the postpericardiotomy syndrome requires the presence of at least 2 of the following: fever lasting beyond the first postoperative week without evidence of infection, pleuritic chest pain, friction rub, evidence of pleural effusion, and evidence of a new or worsening pericardial effusion. It can occur from 3 days up to a year after surgery. Laboratory findings may include a mild leukocytosis and elevated sedimentation rate. Administration of colchicine following coronary bypass grafting for 1 month is safe and efficacious in the prevention of postpericardiotomy syndrome for up to 12 months. It also decreases the rate of disease-related hospitalizations and relapses. Other medications have not been consistently shown to have a similar benefit (answer D is incorrect).

In this example, the physical exam findings do not suggest pericardial tamponade; therefore, proceeding with pericardiocentesis is not appropriate (answer B is incorrect). Since the pleural effusion is small in size, chest tube thoracostomy is also not indicated (answer A is incorrect).

Imazio M, Trinchero R, Brucato A, et al. Colchicine for the prevention of the post-pericardiotomy syndrome (COPPS): a multicentre, randomized, double-blind, placebo-controlled trial. *Eur Heart J* 2010; 31:2749-2754.

74. D. Death is usually due to refractory pulmonary hemorrhage.

SUBJECT: Diffuse alveolar hemorrhage following hematopoietic stem cell transplantation

Diffuse alveolar hemorrhage following hematopoietic stem cell transplantation is defined as evidence of widespread alveolar injury manifested as multilobar infiltrates, signs/symptoms suggestive of pneumonia, abnormal pulmonary physiology showing an increased alveolar to arterial oxygen gradient, and a restrictive ventilatory defect. Infection should be absent. Bronchoalveolar lavage should show a progressively bloodier return or the presence of 20% or more hemosiderin-laden macrophages. Ideally, lavage should be performed in 3 separate subsegmental bronchi to confirm the diagnosis. Biopsy, when performed, will show blood in at least 30% of the alveolar surfaces.

Most cases present within the first month after transplantation although later onset has been described (answer C is a correct statement). Symptoms usually include shortness of breath, cough, and fever. Hemoptysis is typically absent. The incidence is equivalent among autologous and allogenic recipients and is reported to be about 5% (answer A is a correct statement). Risk factors include age greater than 40 years, transplantation for solid tumors, total body irradiation, severe mucositis, renal insufficiency, and fevers. Thrombocytopenia does not appear to be an independent risk factor (answer B is a correct statement). Mortality rates are 80%-100% despite supportive therapy. Death is usually due to sepsis and multisystem organ failure. Respiratory failure from pulmonary hemorrhage is not common. The optimal treatment for diffuse alveolar hemorrhage is unknown.

Kotloff RM, Ahya VN, Crawford SW. Pulmonary complications of solid organ and hematopoietic stem cell transplantation. *Am J Respir Crit Care Med* 2004; 170:22-48.

75. A. *Pseudomonas aeruginosa.*

<u>SUBJECT</u>: Cystic fibrosis and bacterial lung infections

Individuals with cystic fibrosis (CF) have chronic sinopulmonary disease due to persistent colonization with a variety of organisms such as *Staphylococcus aureus*, nontypable *Haemophilus influenzae*, plus mucoid and nonmucoid *Pseudomonas aeruginosa*. Over time one-third of adults will become infected with multidrug resistant gram-negative organisms including *Burkholderia cepacia*, *Stenotrophomonas maltiphilia*, and *Achromobacter xylosoxidans*.

The most common pathogen responsible for pulmonary exacerbations in adults is *P. aeruginosa* (answers B, C, and D are incorrect). Mild exacerbations can be treated with an oral antipseudomonal fluoroquinolone. Moderate to severe exacerbations require treatment with 2 parental antipseudomonal drugs, usually a beta-lactam and an aminoglycoside.

Aerosolized tobramycin has been used successfully to suppress chronic infection. It has been shown to decrease the presence of *P. aeruginosa* in sputum, decrease the number of days of hospitalization, and improve pulmonary function. It should be considered in any patient who is chronically infected with *P. aeruginosa* with an FEV_1 between 25% and 75% of predicted.

There is no convincing evidence to support the routine use of chronic oral antibiotic therapy in individuals with CF. The only possible exception to this is the use of the macrolide azithromycin in individuals > 6 years of age who have persistent *P. aeruginosa* infection. In this select group azithromycin improves the FEV_1 and results in the need for fewer courses of parenteral antibiotics and fewer hospital days. It is unclear how azithromycin exerts a beneficial effect, but it may have to do with anti-inflammatory properties.

Yankaskas JR, Marshall BC, Sufian B, et al. Cystic fibrosis adult care. *Chest* 2004; 125:1S–39S.

76. A. 24 hours.

<u>SUBJECT</u>: Bronchoprovocation testing

Bronchoprovocation testing with methacholine is one method that can be used to assess for airway hyperresponsiveness. It is most useful in excluding a diagnosis of asthma because of the negative predictive power.

There are different dosing protocols for methacholine challenge testing. The 2-minute tidal breathing method and the 5-breath dosimeter method are most commonly used. A PC_{20} (provocative concentration in mg/mL causing a 20% fall in the FEV_1) of < 1.0 is consistent with moderate to severe bronchial hyperresponsiveness, a concentration of 1.0–4.0 with mild bronchial hyperresponsiveness, a concentration of 4.0–16 with borderline bronchial hyperresponsiveness, and a concentration > 16 with normal bronchial hyperresponsiveness.

Absolute contraindications to methacholine challenge testing include the presence of severe airflow limitation (FEV_1 < 50% of predicted), heart attack or stroke in the last 3 months, uncontrolled hypertension (systolic blood pressure > 200 mm Hg or diastolic blood pressure > 100 mm Hg), and known aortic aneurysm. Relative contraindications include moderate air flow limitation (FEV_1 < 60% of predicted), pregnancy, nursing mothers, use of cholinesterase inhibitor medications, and an inability to perform acceptable spirometry.

Medications that decrease bronchial responsiveness should be held prior to testing. Short-acting inhaled bronchodilators should be held for 8 hours, medium-acting bronchodilators (ipratropium) for 24 hours, long-acting inhaled bronchodilators (salmeterol, formoterol) for 48 hours, and tiotropium for 1 week. Intermediate-acting theophyllines should be held for 24 hours and long-acting theophyllines for 48 hours. Leukotriene modifiers should be held for 24 hours. Antihistamines should not be administered for 3 days prior to testing. Foods and beverages that contain caffeine should be withheld on the day of the exam.

Guidelines for methacholine and exercise challenge testing – 1999. *Am J Respir Crit Care Med* 2000; 161:309–329.

77. B. Amlodipine and warfarin.

<u>**SUBJECT**</u>: Pulmonary arterial hypertension

Pulmonary arterial hypertension is defined as a mean pulmonary artery pressure > 25 mm Hg with a pulmonary capillary wedge pressure < 15 mm Hg measured during right heart catheterization. The World Health Organization recognizes several causes of pulmonary arterial hypertension, including the idiopathic form, familial form, in association with collagen vascular diseases, congenital systemic to portal shunts, portal hypertension, infection with the human immunodeficiency virus infection, drugs/toxins, pulmonary venoocclusive disease, and pulmonary capillary hemangiomatosis. Less common causes include hereditary hemorrhagic telangiectasia, splenectomy, and myeloproliferative disorders. The patient in this question has the idiopathic form of pulmonary arterial hypertension.

A vasoreactivity challenge with inhaled nitric oxide, intravenous epoprostenol, or intravenous adenosine resulting in a fall in the mean pulmonary artery pressure > 10 mm Hg to a level < 40 mg Hg with no change or an increase in cardiac output is defined as a positive response. The initial treatment should be with a long-acting calcium channel blocker such as nifedipine, diltiazem, or amlodipine (answers C and D are incorrect). Verapamil should be avoided because of the negative inotropic effects (answer A is incorrect). Anticoagulation should also be simultaneously administered in the absence of a contraindication.

Advanced therapies such as endothelium receptor antagonists, prostanoids, and phosphodiesterase 5 inhibitors should be considered for patients with a negative vasoreactivity test or who fail primary therapy. Patients who are being considered for advanced therapies should be referred to a center with experience in the treatment of pulmonary arterial hypertension.

Badesch DB, Abman SH, Simonneau G, et al. Medical therapy for pulmonary arterial hypertension. *Chest* 2007; 131:1917-1928.

78. C. Magnetic resonance imaging is superior to computed tomography for detecting tumor involvement of the brachial plexus.

SUBJECT: Superior pulmonary sulcus tumor

A superior sulcus tumor arises within the apical pleuropulmonary groove. Such a tumor may result in Pancoast's syndrome, characterized by ipsilateral shoulder/arm pain corresponding to the distribution of the 8th cervical nerve trunk and 1st and 2nd thoracic nerve trunks, Horner's syndrome, and weakness/atrophy of the hand muscles. Horner's syndrome occurs in the majority of patients and is due to invasion of the paravertebral sympathetic chain and the inferior cervical ganglion causing ipsilateral ptosis, myosis, and anhidrosis. Atrophy and weakness of the intrinsic muscles of the hand and pain or paresthesia in the distribution of the ulnar nerve are a result of tumor invasion of C8 and T1 nerve roots.

The majority of cases of Pancoast's tumor are due to non-small cell carcinoma of the lung (answer A is incorrect). Squamous cell carcinoma appears to be more common than adenocarcinoma. Small cell carcinoma is rare. Chest radiographs usually reveal an apical mass. Computed tomography of the chest is helpful to define the extent of the tumor but is not as good as magnetic resonance imaging at identifying chest wall invasion and detecting tumor involvement of surrounding structures such as the subclavian vessels and brachial plexus. Superior sulcus tumors that involve the chest wall are considered T3 lesions. However, once there is involvement of the brachial plexus, mediastinum, or vertebral bodies, the lesion is reclassified as a T4 (answer B is incorrect).

The most common treatment for this tumor is combined preoperative radiotherapy and extensive surgical resection. Five-year survival is estimated to be less than 25% (answer D is incorrect). Contraindications to resection include extensive involvement of the brachial plexus and paraspinal region, mediastinal lymph node involvement, and distant metastasis.

Arcasoy SM, Jett JR. Superior pulmonary sulcus tumors and Pancoast's syndrome. *N Eng J Med* 1997; 337:1370-1376.

79. D. Forced vital capacity less than 65% of predicted.

SUBJECT: Idiopathic pulmonary fibrosis

The patient in this question has idiopathic pulmonary fibrosis (IPF). IPF is defined as a form of chronic, progressive fibrosing interstitial pneumonia of uncertain etiology. The characteristic computed tomography findings are peripheral, subpleural reticular changes with a predilection for the bases. Honeycombing and traction bronchiectasis are present in advanced cases. The key histologic findings are temporal and special heterogeneity with foci of dense fibrosis in a subpleural/paraseptal distribution next to normal-appearing lung. Prognosis is poor with a reported median survival time from 2-3 years following the diagnosis. More recent data suggests that some patients may exceed this survival timeline. The most common cause of death is progressive lung disease.

A number of baseline factors have been shown to be associated with an increased risk of subsequent mortality. The baseline forced vital capacity is of no definite prognostic value. In contrast, a longitudinal change of > 10% from the absolute value may be predictive of mortality. A decline over 6-12 months has also been reliably demonstrated to be associated with a shortened survival. The baseline diffusion capacity for carbon monoxide is a much more reliable predicator for survival with a value < 40% of predicted associated with an increased risk for mortality (answer A is a true statement). A subsequent decline over time by > 15% of the absolute value is also a predicator of poor survival. High-resolution computed tomography features of honeycombing and the presence of pulmonary hypertension (mean pulmonary artery pressure of > 25 mm Hg at rest obtained during right heart catheterization) are also associated with an increased risk of subsequent mortality (answers B and C are true statements).

Raghu G, Collard HR, Egan JJ, et al. An official ATS/ERS/JRS/ALAT statement: Idiopathic pulmonary fibrosis: Evidence-based guidelines for diagnosis and management. *Am J Respir Crit Care Med* 2009; 183:788-824.

80. A. *Schistosoma mansoni.*

<u>SUBJECT</u>: Schistosomiasis

Human schistosomiasis is caused by species of the genus *Schistosoma* (*S. mansoni, S. haematobium, S. japonicum, S. intercalatum, S. mekongi*). The patient in this question was infected with *S. mansoni,* which is endemic in parts of the Middle East such as Egypt and Saudi Arabia. Humans acquire the infection by coming into contact with areas inhabited by the intermediate host, which is a snail. Swimming, bathing, or working in fresh water allows the organism the opportunity to penetrate the skin. This may produce a pruritic rash. The organism then passes through the venous circulation to the pulmonary capillaries. Several weeks later, the individual may experience an acute illness characterized by fever, cough, shortness of breath, diarrhea, arthralgias, chest pain, sweats, and malaise.

The organism then passes into the systemic circulation including venous plexuses within the abdominal cavity and intrahepatic venous system. The latter may ultimately lead to hepatic fibrosis and subsequent cirrhosis. As the worms reproduce within the inferior mesenteric venous plexus, eggs are passed in the feces and urine. Some eggs will also enter into the adjacent venous circulation. If there is significant cirrhosis, eggs in the mesenteric venous plexus will bypass the portal system and, by entering the systemic circulation, embolize to the lungs. Years later, this may result in an obliterative arteriolitis and secondary pulmonary hypertension. Patients may present with clinical manifestations of pulmonary hypertension and cor pulmonale.

Infection with *Plasmodium falciparum* causes malaria (answer D is incorrect). Severe disease may result in noncardiogenic pulmonary edema. *Strongyloides stercoralis* can result in Loeffler's syndrome, which is characterized by transient pulmonary infiltrates and eosinophilia. Clinical symptoms can include cough, dyspnea, and bronchospasm (answer C is incorrect). Infection with *Echinococcus multilocularis* can lead to intrapulmonary fluid-filled cysts (answer B is incorrect).

Bethlem EP, Schettino G, Carvalho C. Pulmonary schistosomiasis. *Curr Opin Pulm Med* 1997; 3:361-365.

81. B. Induce sputum for differential cell count.

<u>SUBJECT</u>: Nonasthmatic eosinophilic bronchitis

Chronic cough is defined as a cough lasting greater than 8 weeks. The most common causes are upper airway syndromes, asthma, and esophageal reflux. Nonasthmatic eosinophilic bronchitis may be the cause in 10%-30% of cases referred to a specialty clinic. The diagnostic work up for chronic cough should focus on the major causes. In this example, upper airway syndromes and asthma have been excluded with appropriate testing, leaving the possibility of esophageal reflux and nonasthmatic eosinophilic bronchitis as potential causes.

The diagnosis of nonasthmatic eosinophilic bronchitis is made by documenting the presence of airway eosinophilia and also clinical improvement in the cough with inhaled glucocorticoids. Airway eosinophilia is confirmed by inducing sputum using nebulized hypertonic saline. A differential cell count analysis with a high eosinophil count (approximately 40%) is supportive of the diagnosis.

If there is a suspicion the chronic cough may be due to esophageal reflux, the preferred diagnostic test is a 24-hour esophageal probe monitor, which is not an option given in this question. Esophagoscopy is not indicated unless there is a concern for esophageal pathology (answer D is incorrect). High-resolution computed tomography of the chest is not routinely performed in the evaluation of chronic cough, especially when chest radiographs are normal (answer C is incorrect). The exception to this is when there is a strong suspicion the patient may have a diffuse parenchymal lung disease or bronchiectasis not appreciated on plain films. Flexible bronchoscopy would be reserved for situations where a diagnosis remains elusive after a thorough evaluation for all other causes has been performed or there is a suspicion that an endobronchial lesion may be present (answer A is incorrect).

Brightling CE. Chronic cough due to nonasthmatic eosinophilic bronchitis. *Chest* 2006; 129:1168-1218.

82. C. Cystic fibrosis.

SUBJECT: Cystic fibrosis epidemiology

Among the Caucasian population in the United States of America, cystic fibrosis (CF) is the most common genetic disease (answers A, B, and D are incorrect). It is an autosomal recessive disorder. The incidence is approximately 1 in 2,000-3,000 births in the Caucasian population. African Americans, Native Americans, Asian Americans, and Hispanic Americans have a much lower incidence.

The CF gene is located on chromosome 7 and encodes for the cystic fibrosis transmembrane regulator (CFTR) protein. This protein is located at the cell surface and functions as an ion channel that regulates chloride secretions. Impairment in the CFTR protein leads to the development of thick secretions in affected organs. A deletion of a single phenylalanine at position 508 is the most common mutation. More than 1,300 mutations of the CFTR gene have been described.

In addition to chronic sinopulmonary disease, other features of CF include gastrointestinal complications such as distal intestinal obstruction syndrome, rectal prolapse, pancreatic insufficiency, and chronic hepatic disease. Complications due to protein calorie malnutrition and fat-soluble vitamin deficiencies may also occur. About 1%–2% of males are fertile with the rest being azoospermic because of abnormalities of the vas deferens. Women may have normal reproductive anatomy.

Yankaskas JR, Marshall BC, Sufian B, et al. Cystic fibrosis adult care. *Chest* 2004; 125:1S–39S.

83. B. Pneumothorax.

SUBJECT: Marfan syndrome

The patient in this question has Marfan syndrome, an autosomal dominant disorder with variable penetrance. The resultant connective tissue abnormalities most commonly affect the cardiovascular system, eyes, and the skeleton. A number of different pulmonary complications have been described in individuals with Marfan syndrome. Spontaneous pneumothorax is the most common complication (answers A, C, and D are incorrect). It can be bilateral and is oftentimes recurrent. Pulmonary bullae, emphysema, bronchiectasis, pneumonia, upper lobe fibrosis, congenital malformations of the middle lobe, and respiratory insufficiency due to chest wall disorders such as pectus excavatum and kyphoscoliosis have also been reported. More recently, it has also been recognized that there is an association with obstructive sleep apnea.

Wood JR, Bellamy D, Child AH, et al. Pulmonary disease in patients with Marfan syndrome. *Thorax* 1984; 39:780–784.

84. C. Theophylline.

SUBJECT: Theophylline toxicity

Theophylline has many clinical indications, including the treatment of asthma and COPD. It appears to exert a bronchodilator effect through inhibition of phosphodiesterase isoenzymes and through epinephrine release. Theophylline may also have anti-inflammatory effects through the inhibition of phosphodiesterase isoenzymes. Other proposed mechanisms of action include an increase in central respiratory drive by adenosine receptor antagonism and an increase in diaphragm muscle contractility through alterations in calcium fluxes.

In patients with COPD, theophylline has been shown to improve the FEV_1, reduce dyspnea, improve exercise tolerance, and increase mucociliary clearance. Theophylline has a narrow therapeutic range. A serum concentration of 10 to 20 mcg/mL is usually targeted although there are data that drug levels of 5-10 mcg/mL may be beneficial. Theophylline serum concentration does not always correlate well with the risk for toxicity. Seizures have been reported with theophylline serum levels as low as 14 mcg/mL. Other signs of toxicity can include nausea, vomiting, abdominal pain, tremor, cardiac arrhythmias, hypotension, hypokalemia, metabolic acidosis, and hyperglycemia. A number of medicines can increase the serum level of theophylline, including the macrolide clarithromycin, which the patient in this question was receiving.

Acute digoxin toxicity presents with nausea, vomiting, anorexia, abdominal distress, and mental status changes (answer A is incorrect). Citalopram toxicity manifests as nausea, tremors, and somnolence. There is a risk for more serious complications such as prolongation of the QTc and serotonin syndrome (answer D is incorrect). Inhaled ipratropium has little risk for toxicity since very little of the drug is absorbed into the systemic circulation (answer B is incorrect).

Vassallo R, Lipsky JJ. Theophylline: Recent advances in the understanding of its mode of action and uses in clinical practice. *Mayo Clin Proc* 1998; 73:346-354.

85. D. In the acquired form, granulocyte macrophage-colony stimulating factor autoantibodies are present.

SUBJECT: Pulmonary alveolar proteinosis

Pulmonary alveolar proteinosis (PAP) is a rare syndrome characterized by the accumulation of surfactant components within the alveoli. The condition can be congenital, acquired, or secondary to some other disorder. The congenital disease is usually attributed to mutations in surfactant protein genes. The acquired form is due to autoantibodies against granulocyte macrophage-colony stimulating factor (GM-CSF) that results in the impairment of surfactant clearance by alveolar macrophages. PAP has also been described in association with several other conditions including exposure to silica, cement dust, aluminum dust, titanium dioxide, as well as immunodeficiency disorders such as severe combined immunodeficiency disorder and immunoglobulin A deficiency. There is also an association with underlying malignancies, although it is not common with solid organ tumors. It occurs almost exclusively with malignancies of hematopoietic origin such as myeloid leukemias (answer A is incorrect).

Acquired PAP typically presents with gradual onset dyspnea, cough, and fatigue that are progressive. The condition is usually present several months before the diagnosis is made. Males are more commonly affected than females. Physical examination may reveal bibasilar crackles, clubbing, and signs of cyanosis. Pulmonary function testing usually shows a restrictive ventilatory defect with reduced diffusion capacity. Laboratory data is generally unremarkable although an elevated lactate dehydrogenase has been described. High-resolution computed tomography scanning usually demonstrates a "crazy-paving" pattern with geographic areas of ground glass opacities with thickening of the interlobular septae. The condition can be successfully diagnosed by examination of bronchoalveolar lavage fluid. The fluid usually contains large amounts of granular acellular eosinophilic proteinaceous material that is periodic acid-shift positive. Biopsy will show near complete filling of the alveolar spaces with acellular surfactant (figures 85-C and 85-D).

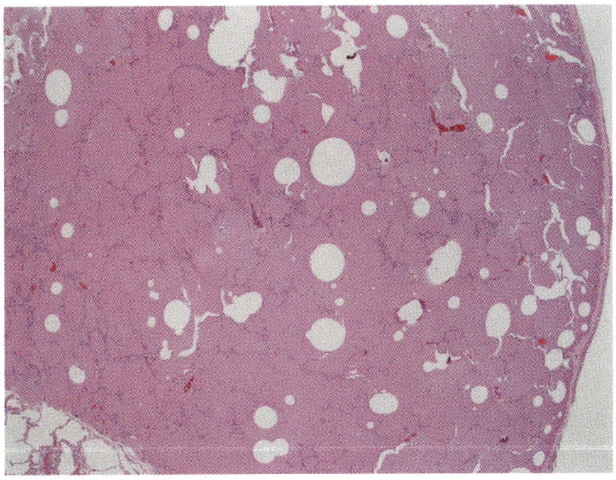

Figure 85-C

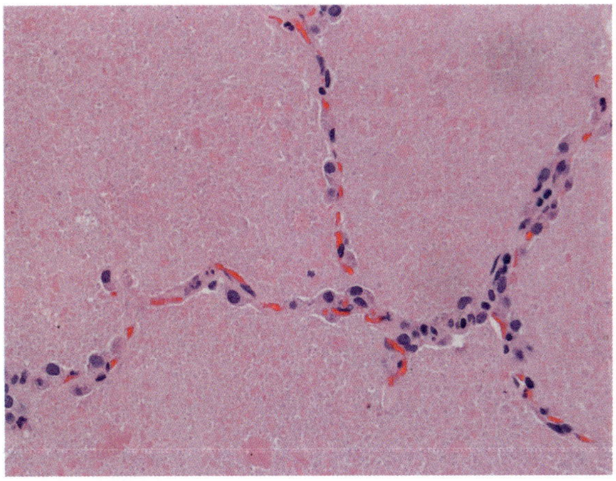

Figure 85-D

Whole lung lavage remains the treatment of choice. This procedure is usually performed in patients who have moderate or severe disease. Patients with mild disease may be successfully observed, and some will eventually experience a spontaneous remission (answer C is incorrect). Of the patients who require whole lung lavage, many will need more than one. Most patients ultimately achieve an extended period of remission. The use of GM-CSF as treatment in patients with acquired PAP is currently undergoing investigation. Patients with PAP are at high risk of secondary infection with pathogens such as atypical mycobacteria, *Aspergillus* spp., *Nocardia* spp., and *Pneumocystis jiroveci.* Antibiotics for prophylaxis against these pathogens, however, are not routinely administered (answer B is incorrect).

Seymour JR, Presneill JJ. Pulmonary alveolar proteinosis. *Am J Respir Crit Care Med* 2002; 166:215-235.

86. B. Doxycycline.

SUBJECT: Q fever

Q fever is caused by *Coxiella brunetti*, a small gram-negative bacterium. Mammals, birds, and ticks are the natural reservoirs. Farm animals such as goats, sheep, and cattle are the most common source of human infection. The bacterium can be aerosolized from newborn animals, the placenta, or contaminated wool. Infection can also be transmitted by consumption of raw milk.

Following infection, there is a highly variable course. The majority of patients are asymptomatic. Some will present with a flu-like syndrome after an incubation period of 2-4 weeks. Fever, relative bradycardia, conjunctivitis, hepatosplenomegaly, and pneumonia may be present. Exanthema, pericarditis, myocarditis, meningitis, encephalitis, hepatitis, and endocarditis may also occur. Chest radiograph findings are nonspecific, but often show a focal pneumonitis. Leukocyte count can be normal. Thrombocytopenia and elevated transaminase levels are commonly observed.

Tetracycline compounds are the recommended treatment for acute Q fever. Doxycycline is the preferred agent (answers A, C, and D are incorrect). Macrolides may be an alternative. Prevention is primarily through avoidance of contact with infected animals.

Raoult D, Marrie T. Q Fever. *Clin Infect Dis* 1995; 20:489-496.

87. A. *Streptococcus pneumoniae.*

SUBJECT: Community-acquired pneumonia

Community-acquired pneumonia (CAP) can be caused by a wide variety of pathogens. In the ambulatory setting, *Stretptococcus pneumoniae* is the most frequently encountered bacterium (answers B, C, and D are incorrect). Other common pathogens include *Mycoplasma pneumoniae*, *Haemophilus influenzae*, and *Chlamydophila pneumoniae*. *Legionella* spp. and respiratory viruses make up a smaller percentage of cases.

CAP due to other pathogens such as *Chlamydophila psittaci*, *Coxiella burnetii*, *Mycobacterium tuberculosis*, influenza, and endemic fungi are largely determined by epidemiologic conditions and host risk factors.

Mandell LA, Wunderink RG, Anzueto A, et al. Infectious Diseases Society of America/American Thoracic Society consensus guidelines on the management of community-acquired pneumonia in adults. *Clin Infect Dis* 2007; 44:S27-72.

88. C. Non-Hodgkin lymphoma.

SUBJECT: Chylothorax

A chylothorax occurs when there is chyle in the pleural space. This is usually due to a disruption or an obstruction of the thoracic duct. The thoracic duct follows the course of the abdominal aorta until the 3rd to 4th thoracic vertebrae. The thoracic duct then moves to the left and continues posteriorly behind the esophagus. The duct terminates at the junction of the left subclavian and left internal jugular veins. The primary function of the thoracic duct is to transport lymph and chyle back into the venous circulation. Disruption or obstruction of the duct above the 5th thoracic vertebrae will result in a left-sided effusion, whereas below this level leads to a right-sided effusion. The majority of effusions are unilateral.

The most common cause of a chylothorax is trauma (which includes surgery). The most common cause of a nontraumatic chylothorax is malignancy with non-Hodgkin lymphoma being the most frequent (answers A, B, and D are incorrect). Other causes of a nontraumatic chylothorax include sarcoidosis, superior vena cava thrombosis, yellow nail syndrome, tuberous sclerosis, lymphangiomyomatosis, and tuberculosis.

The pleural fluid is typically milky in appearance unless the individual has been fasting. The presence of a triglyceride level > 110 mg/dL is suggestive of a chylothorax. The presence of chylomicrons by lipoprotein analysis is diagnostic. The fluid analysis is almost always compatible with an exudate. The cell count will show a predominance of lymphocytes.

Huggins JT. Chylothorax and cholesterol pleural effusion. *Semin Respir Crit Care Med* 2010; 31:743-750.

89. A. A 53-year-old male with a body mass index of 40 kg/m^2.

SUBJECT: Risk assessment for pulmonary complications following noncardiothoracic surgery

Significant risk factors for postoperative pulmonary complications include chronic obstructive pulmonary disease, congestive heart failure, age older than 60 years, smoking, obstructive sleep apnea, American Society of Anesthesiologists Class 2 or greater, serum albumin level < 3.5 g/dL, and functional dependence. Obesity and mild/moderate asthma are not significant risk factors.

A number of surgery specific conditions also place a patient at high risk for postoperative pulmonary complications. These include prolonged surgery (> 3 hours), abdominal surgery, neurosurgery, head and neck surgery, vascular surgery, thoracic surgery, aortic aneurysm repair, general anesthesia, emergency surgery, and use of the neuromuscular blocking agent pancuronium.

The patient in answer B is at risk because of obstructive sleep apnea. The patient in answer C is at risk because of his smoking status. The patient in answer D is at risk because he has chronic obstructive pulmonary disease.

Qaseem A, Snow V, Fritterman N, et al. Risk assessment for and strategies to reduce perioperative pulmonary complications for patients undergoing noncardiothoracic surgery: A guideline from the American College of Physicians. *Ann Intern Med* 2006; 144:575-580.

90. D. Pulmonary artery aneurysm.

SUBJECT: Behçet's disease

Behçet's disease is a systemic disorder that can affect virtually every organ system. The classic triad consists of recurrent oral and genital ulcers and relapsing uveitis. Pulmonary artery aneurysm is the most common form of pulmonary involvement and can range from a single aneurysm to multiple, bilateral aneurysms. Hemoptysis is frequently the presenting symptom. Less common symptoms include chest pain, dyspnea, and cough. Aneurysm rupture is a leading cause of death (answers A, B, and C are incorrect). Other pulmonary manifestations that have been described include pulmonary embolism, in situ thrombus causing pulmonary artery occlusion, pulmonary vasculitis, and pulmonary hemorrhage.

Uzun O, Akpolat T, Erkan L. Pulmonary vasculitis in Behçet disease. *Chest* 2005; 127:2243-2253.

91. B. Thromboendarterectomy.

SUBJECT: Chronic thromboembolic pulmonary hypertension

Following an acute pulmonary embolism, a minority of patients will develop the complication of chronic thromboembolic pulmonary hypertension (CTPH). The exact incidence of this is unknown, but is probably < 1%. Risk factors for CTPH have not been well defined. Antiphospholipid antibodies are identified in 10%-20% of patients, although not all hypercoagulable states appear to predispose to the development of CTPH. While many patients have a known history of venous thromboembolic disease, not all will. The patient in this question had pulmonary emboli following coronary bypass grafting that was misdiagnosed as the postpericardotomy syndrome.

The most common presenting symptom for CPTH is progressive dyspnea. Exertional chest pain, syncope, and lower extremity edema may also be seen. Early in the disease course, physical examination may be unremarkable. With advanced disease, evidence of pulmonary hypertension and cor pulmonale may be present. A characteristic flow murmur over the lung fields that increases with inspiration has also been described. This murmur probably originates from turbulent flow through diseased pulmonary arteries. Diagnostic evaluation should include chest radiography, echocardiography, pulmonary function testing, chest computed tomographic angiography, right heart catheterization, and pulmonary angiography. The finding of thromboembolic occlusion of the pulmonary vasculature must be present to confirm the diagnosis.

The only definitive treatment for CPTH is pulmonary thromboendarterectomy. Only thrombi that are proximal in location are accessible. Potential candidates should be evaluated for the presence of significant hemodynamic impairment, as this may be a contraindication to surgery. Unique postoperative complications include reperfusion pulmonary edema and a "steal" syndrome that is characterized by a redistribution of arterial blood flow away from segments that were previously well perfused into the newly perfused areas. Both of these complications typically resolve, although severe cases can be fatal. Long term, patients are typically maintained on chronic anticoagulation with warfarin.

Pulmonary embolectomy is performed for the treatment of an acute embolism. It is usually reserved for patients with systemic hypotension who have a contraindication to thrombolytics (answer A is incorrect). Suction embolectomy is a technique that uses a catheter to apply negative pressure to remove clot. It can be used in the treatment of acute pulmonary embolism (answer C is incorrect). An inferior vena cava filter is sometimes placed prior to thromboendarterectomy to prevent further emboli during the high-risk perioperative period. Simply placing a filter and administering anticoagulation would not be considered definitive treatment for CPTH (answer D is incorrect).

Piazza G, Goldhaber SZ. Chronic thromboembolic pulmonary hypertension. *N Engl J Med* 2011; 364:351-360.

92. D. The presence of sustained daytime hypoxemia is a prerequisite for the development of diurnal pulmonary hypertension.

SUBJECT: Pulmonary hypertension and obstructive sleep apnea

Obstructive sleep apnea (OSA) is associated with repetitive arterial oxygen desaturation, hypercapnia, large intrathoracic negative pressure swings, and acute increases in pulmonary artery pressure. Early investigations suggested that the repetitive apnea-induced hypoxemia would precipitate vasoconstriction of the pulmonary vasculature leading to permanent pulmonary hypertension. Untreated, this would eventually culminate in cor pulmonale. More recent studies have disproven these conventional beliefs. It is now believed that sustained daytime hypoxemia is a prerequisite for the development of diurnal pulmonary hypertension (answer C is incorrect). Independently, OSA does not appear to lead to cor pulmonale (answer B is incorrect). The degree of daytime hypoxemia is usually explained by conditions such as an underlying chronic cardiopulmonary disorder, or obesity that causes a secondary chest wall restriction and excessive mechanical load.

Trying to estimate the prevalence of pulmonary hypertension in individuals with OSA and no other comorbid conditions has been challenging. Confounding the problem has been the use of liberal definitions of pulmonary hypertension and different means to measure the pulmonary artery pressure. Using a mean pulmonary arterial pressure of 25 mm Hg or greater at rest as measured by right heart catheterization, the prevalence of pulmonary hypertension is reported to be 12%-27%. The degree of pulmonary hypertension is typically mild and generally not clinically evident. The respiratory disturbance index is a weak predicator of the degree of pulmonary hypertension (answer A is incorrect).

Atwood CW Jr., McCrory D, Garcia JG, et al. Pulmonary artery hypertension and sleep-disordered breathing: ACCP evidence-based clinical practice guidelines. *Chest* 2004; 126 (1 Suppl):72S-77S.

93. C. Take a further medication history.

<u>SUBJECT</u>: Aspirin-exacerbated respiratory disease

Aspirin-exacerbated respiratory disease refers to inflammation of the airways resulting in an exacerbation of asthma and rhinitis following the ingestion of aspirin and most other nonsteroidal anti-inflammatory drugs. The condition is commonly referred to as aspirin-induced asthma or the aspirin triad. The patient in this question was taking an over-the-counter aspirin product after running to relieve muscle soreness.

The exact prevalence of aspirin-exacerbated respiratory disease is unknown. The condition is thought to be under diagnosed. It may be present in as many as 10% to 15% of asthmatics. Symptoms usually develop over time in a characteristic pattern: Rhinitis typically appears at an average age of 30 years and becomes increasingly more difficult to treat. Sinusitis, anosmia, and nasal polyposis are usually present. One to five years later, asthma and sensitivity to aspirin develop. After ingestion of aspirin, an asthma attack will typically occur within 3 hours. Rhinorrhea, conjunctival injection, head and neck flushing, and occasionally abdominal discomfort and urticaria occur. The diagnosis should be suspected in cases of chronic nasal congestion and rhinorrhea, nasal polyposis, recurrent sinusitis, and severe attacks of asthma without an apparent trigger. A definitive diagnosis can be made only by provocation testing using increasing doses of aspirin.

To prevent aspirin-exacerbated respiratory disease, cyclooxygenase-1 inhibitors (COX-1) should be avoided. Sodium salicylate and salicylamide can usually be safely ingested. Selective COX-2 inhibitors (for example, celecoxib) are also well tolerated. Acetaminophen is a weak inhibitor of COX-1 and COX-2 and is therefore generally tolerated at low doses. At very high concentrations (doses > 1,000 mg), it can inhibit COX-1. Patients with aspirin-induced respiratory disease can be desensitized to aspirin if necessary. Following desensitization, aspirin can be ingested on a continual basis without respiratory complications.

Short-acting beta agonists and cromoglycates are used to prevent exercise-induced bronchospasm, which the patient in this question does not have (answers A and B are incorrect). Asthmatics should be encouraged to exercise as tolerated. There are data suggesting that inactivity may contribute to poor asthma control (answer D is incorrect).

Szczeklik A, Stevenson DD. Aspirin-induced asthma: Advances in pathogenesis, diagnosis, and management. *J Allergy Clin Immunol* 2003; 111:913-921.

94. C. Relapsing polychondritis.

<u>SUBJECT</u>: Relapsing polychondritis

Relapsing polychondritis is a multisystem disease caused by recurrent episodes of cartilage inflammation and destruction. The ears, nose, and lower respiratory tract are most commonly affected. Subglottic stenosis, tracheal stenosis, and calcification of the trachea with sparing of the posterior membranous wall can be seen. Symptoms of airway involvement can include dyspnea, cough, strider, and hoarseness. There is no involvement of the lung parenchyma or pulmonary vasculature. Nonerosive seronegative arthritis, ocular inflammation, and vestibular disease may also be present. Approximately one-third of patients with relapsing polychondritis will have a coexisting autoimmune disease such as rheumatoid arthritis, systemic lupus erythematosus, or Sjögren's syndrome.

The most common radiologic finding is anterior airway wall thickening with or without calcification. Tracheobronchomalacia may also be seen. In the presence of airway involvement, pulmonary function tests will show an abnormal shape to the flow volume loop suggesting an obstruction. Patterns of fixed obstruction, variable extrathoracic obstruction, and variable intrathoracic obstruction have all been described depending on the location of the lesion.

Bronchoscopy is often performed in patients experiencing respiratory symptoms. The most common finding is tracheobronchomalacia followed by subglottic stenosis. The patient in this question has subglottic stenosis, evident by stridor on exam and the radiographic appearance of the trachea. A variety of endoscopic interventions are available for treatment of subglottic stenosis including endobronchial laser therapy, balloon dilation, airway stenting, and tracheostomy.

The other disorders given as options in this question are not associated with subglottic stenosis. Giant cell arteritis is a vasculitis that involves medium and large-size vessels. It is characterized by headache, jaw claudication, and visual changes. Pulmonary manifestations are not common, although cough and pulmonary artery aneurysm have been reported (answer A is incorrect). Bechet's is also a systemic vasculitis characterized by recurrent oral ulcers. Pulmonary complications include venous thromboembolism, diffuse alveolar hemorrhage, and pulmonary artery aneurysm formation (answer B is incorrect). Rheumatoid arthritis is a systemic, inflammatory disorder mainly involving the joints. Pulmonary manifestations include interstitial lung disease, organizing pneumonia, and pleural disease (answer D is incorrect).

Rafeq S, Trentham D, Ernst A. Pulmonary manifestations of relapsing polychondritis. *Clin Chest Med* 2010; 31:513-518.

95. B. Prescribe azithromycin.

<u>**SUBJECT**</u>: Pertussis

Bordetella pertussis is a gram-negative coccobacillus that is highly contagious and causes an acute respiratory illness. The incubation period is typically 1 to 3 weeks. Pertussis usually follows 3 phases. The catarrhal phase consists of coryza, conjunctival irritation, and mild cough. A mild temperature elevation can also be seen. Approximately 7 to 10 days later, the paroxysmal phase begins, characterized by the onset of a worsening cough. The cough can be triggered by activities such as exertion and laughter. Complications from coughing such as syncope, urinary incontinence, and emesis can occur. The patient in this question developed a subconjunctival hemorrhage from coughing. The paroxysmal phase may last several weeks. The convalescent phase is characterized by a gradual waning of the cough.

Patients evaluated during the first 3 weeks after cough onset should undergo diagnostic testing with culture and polymerase chain reaction (PCR) assay. A positive culture of nasopharyngeal secretions is considered the gold standard for the diagnosis of pertussis. PCR assay is also helpful as it can test for both viable and nonviable organisms. Serologic testing should be considered for patients who have been coughing longer than 4 weeks.

Antibiotics should be administered during the first 4 weeks of the illness. Antibiotics hasten clearance of the organism and reduce the risk of transmitting the infection. Individuals who are health care workers, or may come in contact with infants or women in the 3rd trimester of pregnancy, should be treated even 6 to 8 weeks after the onset of the illness. The newer macrolide antibiotics (azithromycin and clarithromycin) are first line agents. Trimethoprim-sulfamethoxazole is an alternative antibiotic. Vaccination remains the primary method of disease prevention.

There are no proven therapies to reduce the cough associated with pertussis. Ipratropium is an anticholinergic agent. Oral ipratropium is indicated for bronchospasm associated with COPD and the treatment of acute asthma exacerbations (answer C is incorrect). Nasal ipratropium is indicated for treatment of rhinorrhea associated with the common cold and allergic rhinitis (answer D is incorrect). A combination of a first-generation antihistamine and decongestant is indicated for the relief of rhinitis symptoms due to allergies (answer A is incorrect).

Hewlett EL, Edwards KM. Pertussis – Not just for kids. *N Engl J Med* 2005; 352:1215-1222.

96. D. The tumor originates on the parietal pleura and spreads to the visceral pleura.

SUBJECT: Malignant mesothelioma

Individuals at greatest risk for malignant pleural mesothelioma are those with a history of significant asbestos exposure. There is a dose-dependent relationship between asbestos exposure and the risk of developing mesothelioma. Unlike with bronchogenic carcinoma, cigarette smoking is not associated with mesothelioma (answer A is incorrect). The mean age at the time of presentation is about 60 years. This is due to the long latency period, sometimes 30 to 40 years, from the time of asbestos exposure.

Although this tumor can develop on peritoneal and pericardial surfaces, most are pleural based. The tumor starts on the parietal pleural and spreads to the visceral pleural. Chest radiographs typically show a unilateral pleural effusion. It is more common on the right than the left side. If extensive pleural thickening is present, ipsilateral shift of the mediastinum may be seen. Presenting symptoms usually include nonpleuritic chest pain, shortness of breath, and cough. A number of paraneoplastic syndromes have been described with malignant mesothelioma, including thrombocytosis, hemolytic anemia, hypoglycemia, and hypercalcemia.

The prognosis for malignant mesothelioma remains poor. The median survival from the time of diagnosis is usually 6-18 months. Epithelioid subtype, which the patient in this question has, is the most common tumor and has a better prognosis than sarcomatous cell type (answer B is incorrect). Younger age and better performance status are also favorable prognostic variables. Although metastasis to extrathoracic sites can occur, most patients will die from complications of local tumor invasion and respiratory failure (answer C is incorrect).

Antman, KH. Natural history and epidemiology of malignant mesothelioma. *Chest* 1993; 103:373S–376S.

97. C. Embolization.

SUBJECT: Pulmonary arteriovenous malformations

Pulmonary arteriovenous malformations (PAVM) represent an abnormal communication between a pulmonary artery and a pulmonary vein. Most are congenital, with the majority occurring in the presence of hereditary hemorrhagic telangiectasia (HHT). HHT is an autosomal dominant condition characterized by cutaneous and visceral arteriovenous malformations. Less common causes of PAVM include hepatic cirrhosis, schistosomiasis, and metastatic thyroid carcinoma.

Congenital PAVMs, when severe, may manifest early in life as cyanosis and congestive heart failure. It is more typical, however, for symptoms to occur between the 4th and 6th decades. The most common respiratory complaint is dyspnea that is worse when the individual is sitting or standing and relieved in a recumbent position (platypnea). The objective correlate to this is orthodeoxia, a decrease in the PaO_2 or SaO_2 upon assuming a seated or upright position. Platypnea-orthodeoxia is the result of an increase in blood flow through a PAVM. The second most common respiratory symptom is hemoptysis. Physical examination frequently shows clubbing and manifestations of cyanosis. Individuals with HHT may have cutaneous telangiectasias present.

Chest radiography and chest computed tomography often demonstrate the classic PAVM appearance of a round mass with a uniform density typically in the lower lobes. Multiple lesions may be present. A characteristic feature is the presence of feeding vessels. Contrast echocardiography is a valuable diagnostic tool to look for intrapulmonary shunt physiology. With a PAVM, contrast should be evident in the left atrium after a delay of 3–8 cardiac cycles because of the time required to cross the pulmonary vasculature. In contrast, an intracardiac shunt is usually evident within one cardiac cycle. Pulmonary angiography is considered the gold standard for the diagnosis of PAVM. PAVM is associated with significant morbidity and mortality. Left untreated, PAVM has an incidence of stroke that approximates 11% and brain abscess 7%. Other complications include seizure, migraine headaches, life-threatening hemoptysis, polycythemia, and infectious endocarditis.

It is recommended that symptomatic PAVMs, and those > 2 cm in diameter, be treated. It has also been suggested that a PAVM of < 2 cm in diameter with a feeding artery > 3 mm in diameter be considered for treatment because of the risk of paradoxical embolism. Historically, surgery with definitive resection of the PAVM was the only treatment choice available. Surgery, however, can be associated with significant morbidity and is not practical in an individual with multiple, bilateral lesions. Embolization therapy is now commonly performed. This involves localization of the PAVM by angiography and selective catheterization of the feeding artery. Occlusion of the feeding artery is performed using embolic material such as stainless steel coils. This procedure is associated with a low risk for complications. Pleuritic chest pain, pulmonary infarction, and air embolism can all occur. Individuals with PAVM should receive prophylactic antibiotic therapy before dental and surgical procedures to reduce the risk of cerebral abscess.

There is no established role for the use of pharmacologic therapy in the treatment of PAVM (answers A, B, and D are incorrect). In individuals with HHT, a number of drug therapies have been used to control bleeding. High dose estrogens have been used to control gastrointestinal bleeding. The antiestrogen tamoxifen has been reported to reduce the incidence of epistaxis. Bevacizumab, an angiogenesis inhibitor, has shown promise in the treatment of hepatic AVM and hepatic failure.

Gossage JR, Kani G. Pulmonary arteriovenous malformation. *Am J Respir Crit Care Med* 1998; 158:643-661.

98. C. Observation.

SUBJECT: Acute bronchitis

Acute bronchitis is manifested predominantly by a cough lasting no more than 3 weeks. The cough may or may not be productive of sputum. The diagnosis of acute bronchitis should not be made unless other conditions that can produce acute cough such as asthma, exacerbation of COPD, and pneumonia have been excluded. Chest radiographs are not required unless there are physical examination findings suggesting pneumonia, such as temperature > 38.0 °C, heart rate > 100 beats/min, respiratory rate > 24 breaths/min, bronchial breath sounds, region of dullness to percussion, or crackles.

Acute bronchitis is considered a self-limited illness, and therefore observation is usually all that is necessary. Routine treatment with antibiotics is not justifiable (answer A is incorrect). $Beta_2$ agonist bronchodilators should not be routinely used but may be beneficial in selected patients who have pronounced wheezing (answer B is incorrect). There are no data to suggest a benefit to mucokinetic agents (answer D is incorrect). The use of codeine or dextromethorphan to reduce cough frequency has not been rigorously studied. Because these agents can be effective in patients with chronic bronchitis, it may be reasonable to offer an empiric trial for severe coughing during an episode of acute bronchitis.

Respiratory viruses are the most common cause of acute bronchitis. Common pathogens include coronavirus, rhinovirus, adenovirus, influenza A/B, and respiratory syncytial virus. Bacteria are unlikely to produce acute bronchitis in previously healthy adults; however, if the course is complicated, *Bordetella pertussis* should be excluded.

Braman, SS. Chronic cough due to acute bronchitis: ACCP evidence-based clinical practice guidelines. *Chest* 2006; 129:95S-103S.

99. A. The majority of pneumothoraces occur on the right side.

SUBJECT: Catamenial pneumothorax

Catamenial pneumothorax is defined as a spontaneous pneumothorax occurring within 72 hours before or after the onset of menstruation. It is thought to be the most common clinical manifestation of intrathoracic endometriosis. Catamenial hemothorax, catamenial hemoptysis, and pulmonary nodules are the other manifestations. Approximately two-thirds of patients with catamenial pneumothorax will have pelvic endometriosis. This patient's history of low back pain, constipation, and abdominal bloating are symptoms of pelvic endometriosis.

Catamenial pneumothorax occurs predominantly on the right side. While the exact pathophysiology is unclear, it is believed that there is migration of endometrial tissue from the peritoneal cavity into the pleural space. This can occur through transdiaphragmatic lymphatic channels, hematogenous spread, or diaphragmatic fenestrations. The shedding of endometrial tissue that occurs with menstruation results in pleural irritation and potentially a pneumothorax.

Treatment with hormonal therapy that suppresses ovarian secretion of estrogen is effective in about 50% of cases. Definitive treatment for catamenial pneumothorax is thoracoscopic surgery with stapling of any blebs, closure of diaphragmatic defects, and pleurodesis.

Answers B and C can be seen with lymphangiomyomatosis. Answer D represents cutaneous manifestations of tuberous sclerosis.

Peikert T, Gillespie DJ, Cassivi SD. Catamenial pneumothorax. *Mayo Clin Proc* 2005; 80:677-680.

100. C. Liver transplantation.

<u>SUBJECT</u>: Hepatopulmonary syndrome

Diagnostic criteria for the hepatopulmonary syndrome (HPS) include an oxygen defect (partial pressure of oxygen < 80 mm Hg or alveolar-arterial oxygen gradient > 15 mm Hg while breathing ambient air), pulmonary vascular dilatation, and the presence of liver disease. Any acute or chronic form of liver disease can lead to HPS. Preexisting portal hypertension is not necessary for the development of HPS. There is not a linear relationship between the severity of liver disease and the clinical manifestations of HPS.

The vascular defect of HPS is dilated pulmonary capillaries, which can be focal or diffuse. Less commonly, arterial venous communications are present. The most useful method to detect pulmonary vascular dilation is contrast enhanced transthoracic echocardiography with saline injection. Microbubble opacification of the left atrium within 3 to 8 cardiac cycles indicates passage through an abnormally dilated vascular bed. Transesophageal contrast echocardiography to look for an atrial septal defect can be performed if there is a suspicion of a right to left cardiac shunt. Pulmonary angiography is typically not performed unless there is evidence to support an arterial venous communication that would be amendable to embolization.

There is no proven effective medical treatment for HPS. Transjugular intrahepatic portosystemic shunt has been used in some cases with variable outcomes. It is not recommended as a primary therapy (answer D is incorrect). Inhaled nitric oxide is a pulmonary vasodilator that is used for acute vasodilator testing in the evaluation of adults with pulmonary arterial hypertension (answer A is incorrect). Propanolol is a nonselective beta-blocker that has been used for prophylaxis of variceal bleeding in individuals with cirrhosis, but has not been shown to be of therapeutic benefit for HPS (answer B is incorrect). Liver transplantation remains the only proven treatment. This leads to the spontaneous resolution of HPS. The time course for resolution of hypoxemia is highly variable, with some individuals improving quickly over days and others gradually improving over months.

Rodrigues-Roisin R, Korwka MJ. Hepatopulmonary syndrome – A liver-induced lung vascular disorder. *N Engl J Med* 2008; 358:2378–2387.

LABORATORY REFERENCE VALUES AND ABBREVIATIONS

Hematologic

CD4 lymphocyte count	500-1550/cu mm
D-dimer	< 200 ng/mL
Erythrocyte sedimentation rate (Westergren)	Female: 0-25 mm/hr; male: 0-20 mm/hr
Hematocrit	Female: 39-47%; male: 41-49%
Hemoglobin	Female: 12-15 g/dL; male: 13-16 g/dL
Leukocyte count and differential	Leukocyte count: 4,500-11,000/cu mm 50-70% segmented neutrophils 0-5% band forms 0-3% eosinophils 0-1% basophils 30-45% lymphocytes 0-6% monocytes
Mean corpuscular volume (MCV)	85-97 fL
Partial thromboplastin time	25-40 seconds
Platelet count	150,000-350,000/cu mm
Prothrombin time	11-14 seconds

Whole blood, plasma, serum chemistries

Albumin	3.6-5.5 g/dL
Aldolase	0.9-3.0 IU/mL

Alkaline phosphatase	40–125 U/L
$Alpha_1$-antitrypsin (AAT)	20–55 micromol/L
Aminotransferase, serum alanine (ALT)	15–40 U/L
Aminotransferase, serum aspartate (AST)	15–40 U/L
Amylase	30–125 U/L
Antibodies to double-stranded DNA	< 25% DNA-bound
Anticardiolipin antibodies	IgG: > 20 GPL units is positive
Antimitrochondrial antibodies	> 1:5 is abnormal
Antinuclear antibody (ANA)	> 1:45 is abnormal
Antinuclear cytoplasmic antibody (ANCA) cytoplasmic (c-ANCA) perinuclear (p-ANCA)	< 1:20
Antistreptolysin O titer	< 205 Todd units
Arterial studies (room air) PaO_2 $PaCO_2$ Bicarbonate pH Oxygen saturation	 75–100 mm Hg 37–42 mm Hg 24–27 mEq/L 7.36–7.45 ≥ 95%
Bilirubin, total	0.4–1.0 mg/dL
Blood urea nitrogen (BUN)	8–19 mg/dL
Brain natriuretic peptide	< 170 pg/mL
Complement C3 C4	 110–230 mg/dL 15–50 mg/dL
Creatinine kinase Total MB isoenzymes	 5–50 U/L < 5% of total
Creatinine	0.6–1.3 mg/dL
Digoxin	0.9–2.0 ng/mL

Electrolyes Sodium Potassium Chloride Bicarbonate	 135-144 mEq/L 3.4-5.0 mEq/L 98-105 mEq/L 24-28 mEq/L
Glucose	Normal (fasting): 70-115 mg/dL
IgE	< 400 IU/mL
Lactate dehydrogenase (LDH)	135-270 U/L
Protein, total	5.4-8.9 g/dL
Rheumatoid factor	> 1:80 is abnormal
Theophylline	7-20 mcg/mL

38138730R00093

Made in the USA
Lexington, KY
23 December 2014